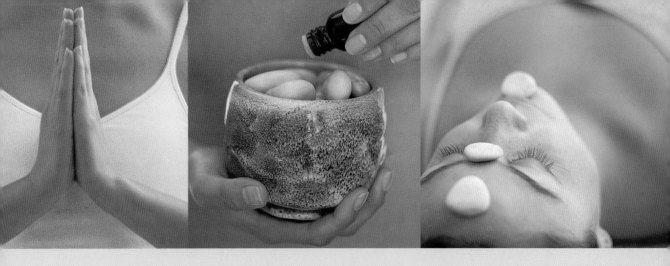

The Body Shop

BodyCare
Manual

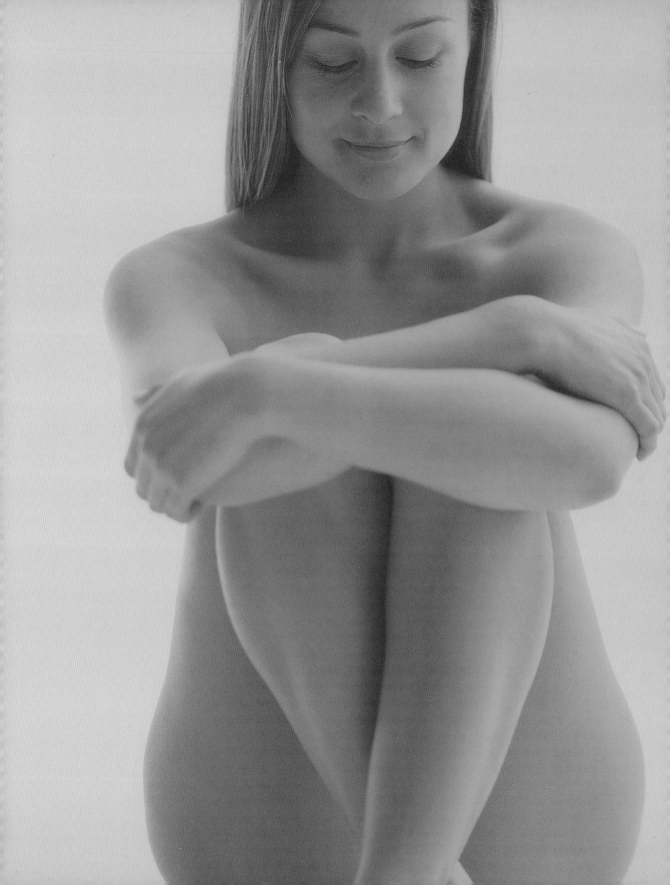

The Body Shop
BodyCare
Manual

BY Mona Behan
AND Susan Elisabeth Davis
PHOTOGRAPHY BY John Robbins
FOREWORD BY Justine Roddick

BARNES
& NOBLE
BOOKS
NEW YORK

This edition published by Barnes & Noble, Inc.
by arrangement with Weldon Owen Inc.

2003 Barnes & Noble Books
Copyright © 2003 Weldon Owen Inc.

THE BODY SHOP INTERNATIONAL, PLC
Founder Anita Roddick
Chairman Adrian Bellamy
Chief Executive Officer Peter Saunders
Director of Product Caroline Hadfield
Publications Manager Justine Roddick

WELDON OWEN INC.
Chief Executive Officer John Owen
Chief Operating Officer and President Terry Newell
Vice President and Publisher Roger Shaw
Vice President, International Sales Stuart Laurence

Publisher Rebecca Poole Forée
Creative Director Gaye Allen
Senior Art Director Emma Boys
Business Manager Richard Van Oosterhout
Production Director Chris Hemesath
Color Manager Teri Bell
Production Coordinator Libby Temple

Designer Leon Yu
Managing Editor Elizabeth Dougherty
Make-up Artists Alisha Meek, Olaf Derlig
Stylists Nicole Peters, Yael Gitai
Copy Editor Cynthia Rubin
Recipe Consultant Jennifer Newens
Researchers Kathy P. Behan, Juli Vendzules
Proofreaders Tom Hassett, Katherine L. Kaiser
Indexer Ken DellaPenta

"The Body Shop" and the "Pod" device are registered
trademarks of The Body Shop International, PLC, UK.

A catalog record for this book is available from the
Library of Congress, Washington, D.C.

First printed in 2003

M 10 9 8 7 6 5 4 3 2 1

ISBN 0-7607-5285-0

Set in Bembo™ and Benton Gothic™
Color separations by Bright Arts Hong Kong
Printed in China by Midas Printing Limited

A Note about This Book

This book was printed using soy-based inks on
totally chlorine-free (TCF) paper consisting of
50 percent recycled fibers. The book is bound with
nontoxic glue made from nonanimal sources.

Disclaimer

This book is not intended as a medical
reference guide. The advice contained is
not to be construed as medical diagnosis
or treatment, and should not be used as a
substitute for the advice of qualified health
practitioners. Neither The Body Shop, nor
the publisher, nor the authors can be held
responsible for adverse reactions, damage,
or injury resulting from the use of the
content herein. Any practice of massage,
spa treatments, aromatherapy, yoga, tai chi,
or other suggestions contained herein is
done at the reader's sole discretion and risk.
During pregnancy or for serious or long-term
medical conditions, consult a qualified
health practitioner before engaging in any
treatments or exercises, consuming featured
foods or drinks, or using aromatherapy.

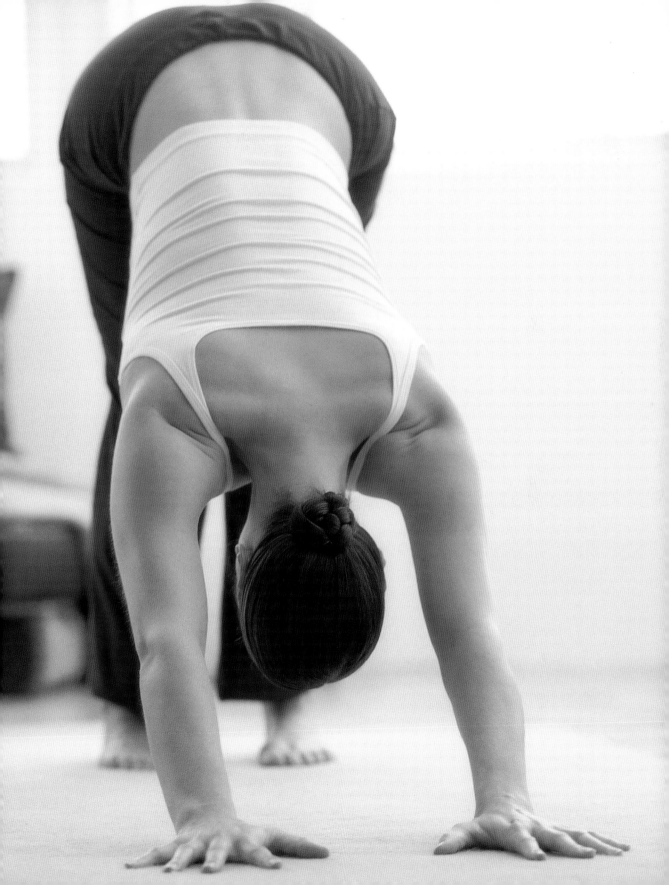

contents

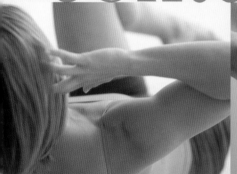

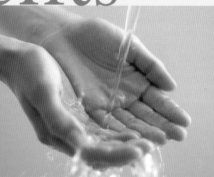

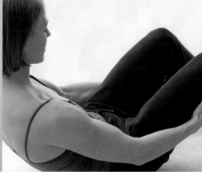

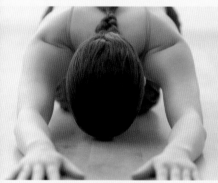

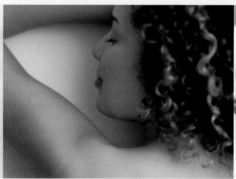

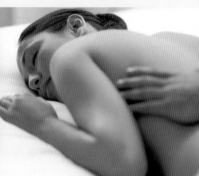

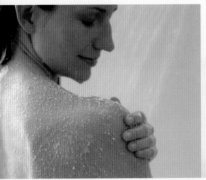

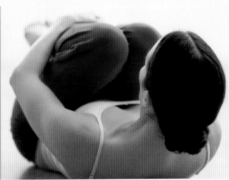

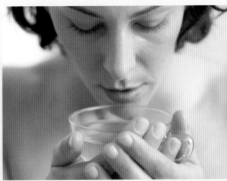

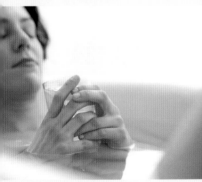

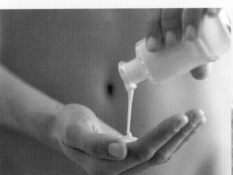

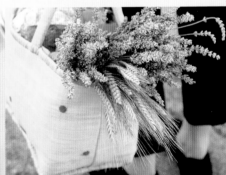

treatments and activities

skin care, hair care, and spa

aromatherapy

massage

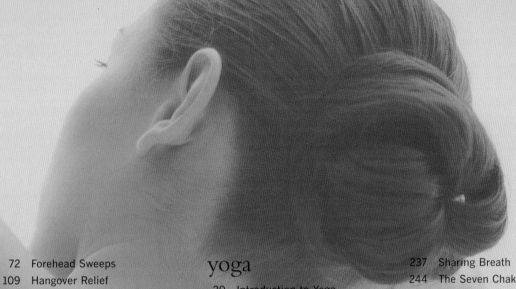

treatments and activities

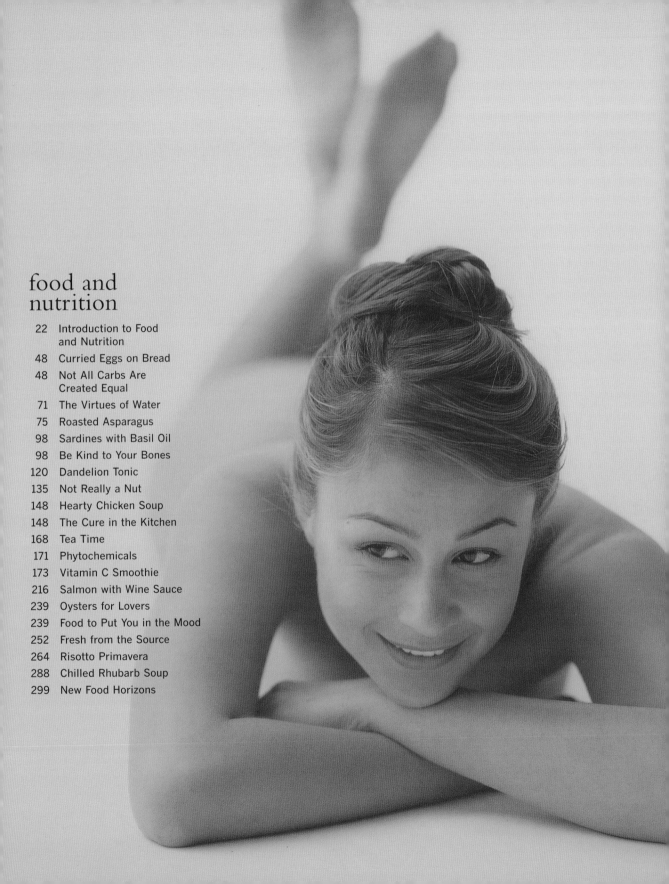

food and
nutrition

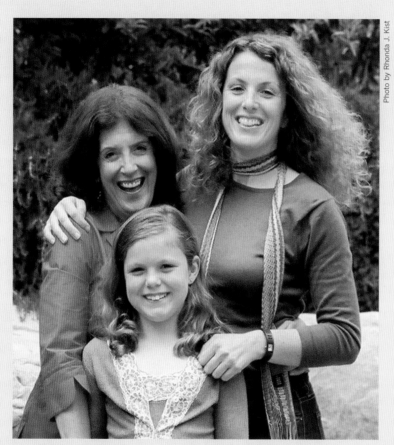

Dame Anita Roddick, Maiya Roddick-Fuller, and Justine Roddick (left to right)

foreword

When my parents, Anita and Gordon Roddick, founded The Body Shop about 30 years ago, they set out to create a different kind of cosmetics company. Far from pushing women into trying to attain some unrealistic, narrow ideal, they expanded the notion of beauty to include all body types, all ages, and all races and ethnicities. They drew inspiration and knowledge from traditional cultures from around the world, concentrated on natural ingredients, and encouraged women to "love their bodies" even if they would never be mistaken for runway models.

My parents also believed that the concept of beauty includes a healthy body, a keen mind, and a good sense of self-esteem. They incorporated this emphasis on wellbeing into The Body Shop's philosophy and raised my sister and me with these ideals as well. I consider it an invaluable legacy that I am trying to pass along to my daughter, Maiya.

You'll see this holistic approach toward beauty and wellbeing reflected in this book. It affected everything from the types of wide-ranging activities we included to the types of strong, healthy women we photographed. We hope you'll find *The Body Shop Body Care Manual* a source of great inspiration, information, and empowerment—one that you'll turn to again and again on your own quest for physical and mental wellbeing.

Justine Roddick

wellbeing

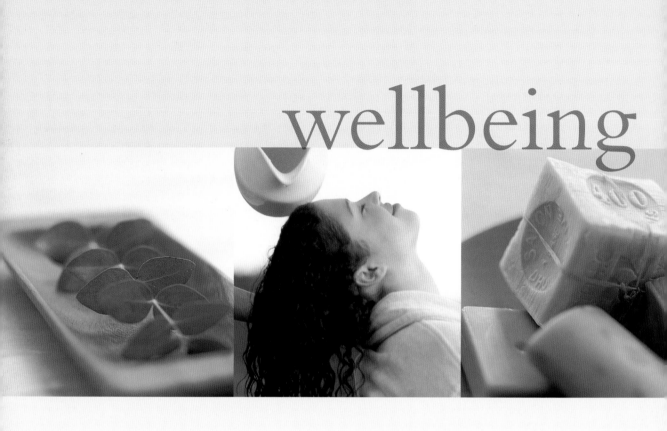

The very word is a promise of the good life.
Not in the materialistic sense, but in the sense of
a life well lived—in a state of contentment,
robust health, and mental vigor.

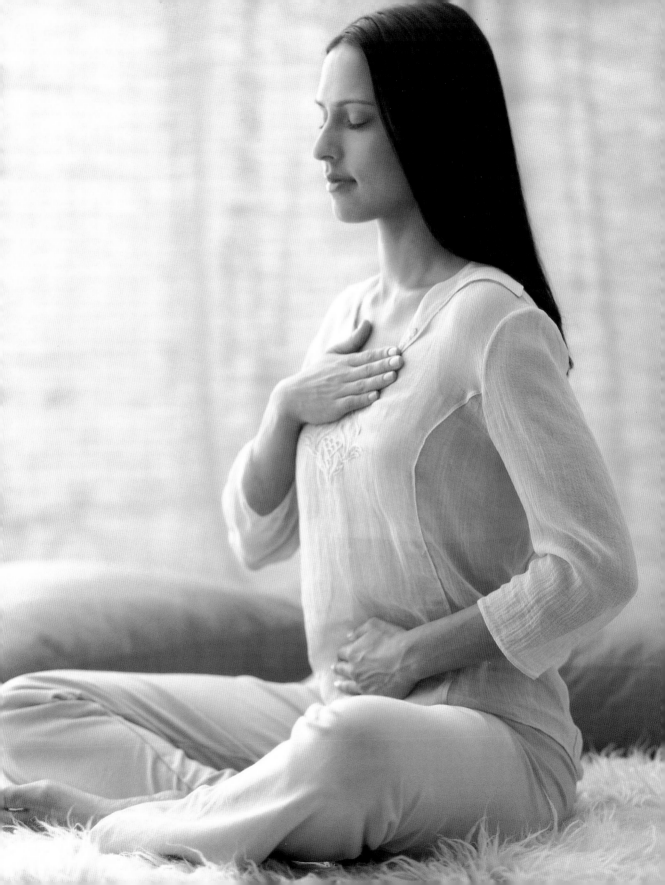

For most women, wellbeing is an ideal we strive to impart to others—our children, our partners, our friends and relatives. But sometimes women need to make a concerted effort to attend to our own wellbeing, to nurture the nurturer. That's where this book comes in. On these pages, you'll find hundreds of imaginative, practical ideas for enhancing your health, outlook, and appearance. These ideas were drawn from a variety of fields, everything from aromatherapy to yoga, from massage to nutrition, and are organized thematically to help you attain specific benefits, such as renewed energy, a stronger body, a state of blissful relaxation, or a little well-earned pampering. The approach is holistic—the needs of the body, mind, and spirit are addressed—and the activities, all contributed by experts in their fields, combine the best of time-honored, traditional disciplines with the latest scientific findings. With its breadth of exercises and its inspirational, informative approach, *The Body Shop Body Care Manual* is your essential guide to wellbeing.

The activities that we describe here will give you a taste of many treatments and traditions: skin care, hair care, spa treatments, aromatherapy, massage, yoga, meditation, breathing techniques, Pilates, tai chi, general fitness, and nutrition. The exercises are designed for beginners, but the descriptions aren't meant to be treatises on the subject. Our hope is that these tastes will help you identify some new fields that interest you and lead you to investigate them further, whether it's through classes, books, or videos. Read *The Body Shop Body Care Manual* from beginning to end, or just start by looking for the chapters that most spark your interest—whether it's learning new ways to unwind, new ways to prevent illness, or new reasons to treat yourself with a little more care.

Here are brief synopses of the treatments and traditions we cover:

skin care, hair care, and spa

The world of beauty has long been the domain of women and has long been filled with all sorts of wonderful (and sometimes not-so-wonderful) tips that are passed from mother to daughter, friend to friend, and beautician to client. Throughout the 20th century, and even today, some beauty products have become increasingly laden with chemicals and oriented toward covering, rather than enhancing, our features. But these days, numerous simple, natural products are also available

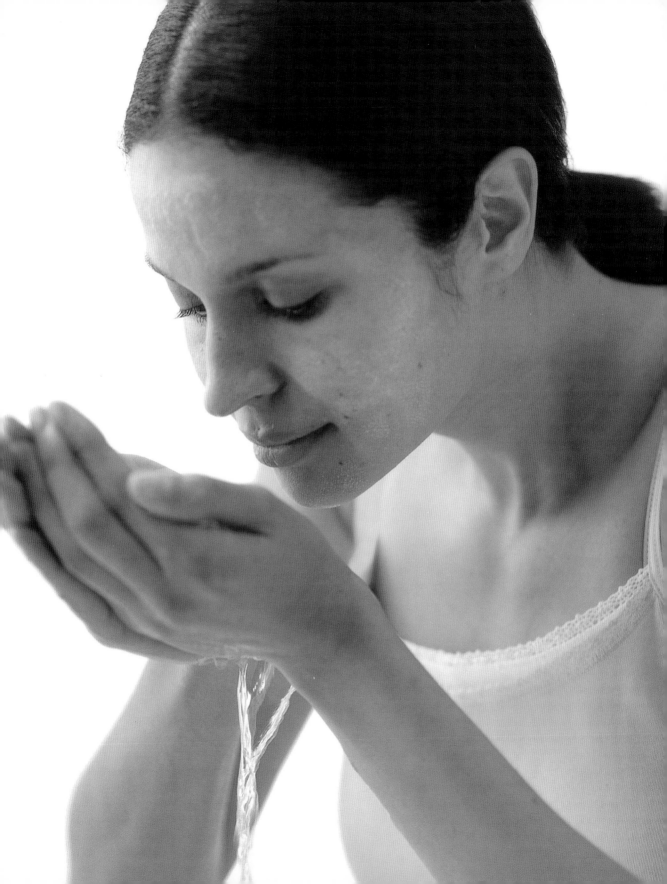

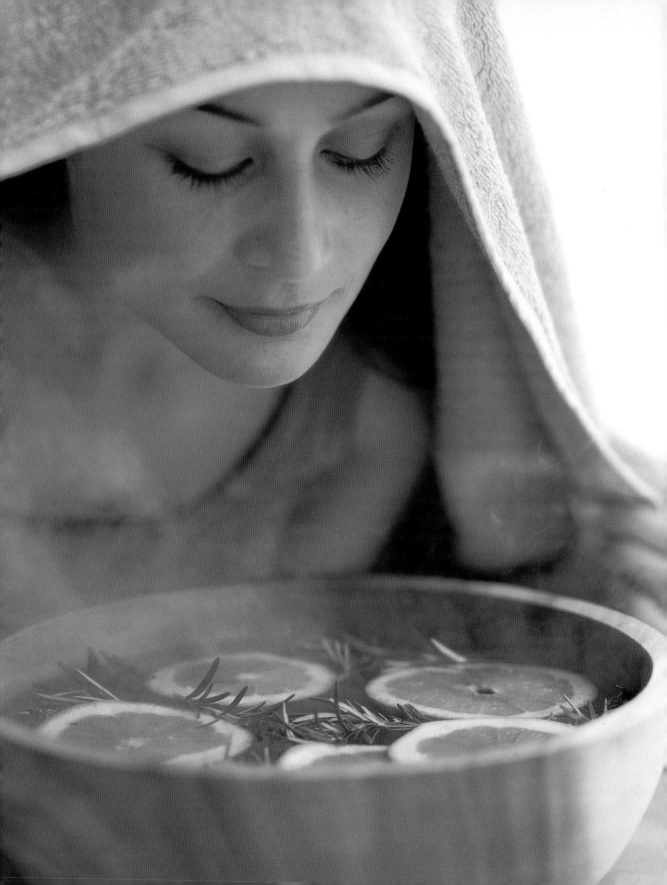

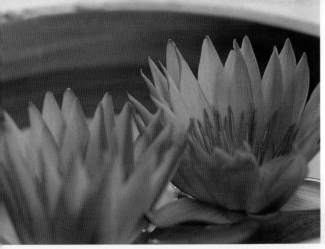
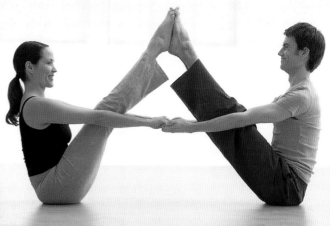

to make you look and feel your best. The greatest beauty secret of all? You can do many of the treatments in just a few minutes in the privacy of your home, as you'll see in the suggestions we offer in the following pages.

aromatherapy

The use of essential oils (oils distilled from aromatic plants) to promote physical, emotional, and spiritual health dates back at least 6,000 years. Today, essential oils are used in a number of ways—in massage oils and body lotions, dispersed in the bath, and diffused in the air. Available in health and beauty stores, as well as on the Internet, essential oils are used to treat a range of maladies and conditions, including stress, depression, headaches, anxiety, menstrual discomfort, and skin problems. While some say that anything that smells good will make you feel good, recent scientific research has shown that aromatherapy truly has health benefits.

massage

In today's fast-paced, individualistic world, one crucial lesson is often forgotten: Humans need touch, and touch is a powerful healer. Indeed, for thousands of years, many cultures have practiced some form of massage with the aim of easing physical, mental, and spiritual ailments. That's not simply the stuff of folklore— research shows us again and again that touch can help reduce stress hormones, alleviate depression, boost the immune system, and diminish pain. And effective massages don't have to come only from certified massage therapists. Simple massages—like those we've chosen here—can also be exchanged at home between lovers, friends, and family members, as well as administered to oneself.

yoga, meditation, and breathing

In Sanskrit (the ancient language of the elite Indian Brahmins), *yoga* means "union," or an integration of body, mind, and spirit. While yoga originated 5,000 years ago in India, the practice is now extremely popular throughout the world, with everyone from schoolchildren to film stars lining up for classes. The discipline consists of a series of poses (called *asanas*), breathing exercises (*pranayama*), and meditation techniques, all of which improve health, strength, and flexibility, as well as help us find inner peace. Of the many types of yoga, we have chosen to focus on hatha yoga, which strives to unite energizing and relaxing body energies. You'll also find breathing techniques that are helpful while doing yoga poses or when simply used on their own, as well as general meditation exercises, such as creative visualization, which involve systematically focusing the mind on a regular basis to achieve clarity and a sense of calm.

pilates

This exercise regimen, which was developed by German dancer and boxer Joseph Pilates (puh-LAH-tees) in the 1920s, is becoming increasingly popular because it helps improve posture, enhance flexibility, and develop strong muscles, especially those of the abdomen, back, and buttocks. Unlike weight training, Pilates elongates muscles, which gives the body a long, lean look. In addition, Pilates emphasizes the importance of developing a strong mind–body connection and incorporates breathing techniques into the exercises. That promised combination of concentration, flexibility, and strength has proven enormously attractive to dancers and actors— as well as athletes, businesspeople, suburban moms, and students the world over.

tai chi

An ancient martial art that originated in China, tai chi (pronounced tie-CHEE) is also known as Chinese shadow boxing. Now it is used as both a fighting and a healing technique, as well as a form of moving meditation. In Chinese, *tai* means "great" and *chi* means "energy," and the practice is all about experiencing, strengthening, and enhancing the flow of life energy in the body. Tai chi consists of a series of slow, graceful, and, ultimately, very powerful movements that involve

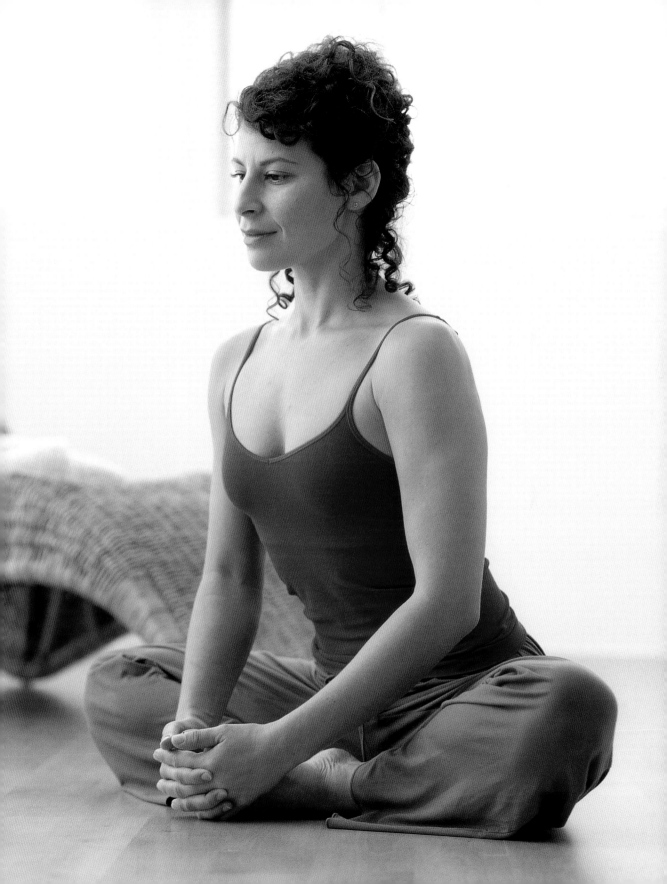

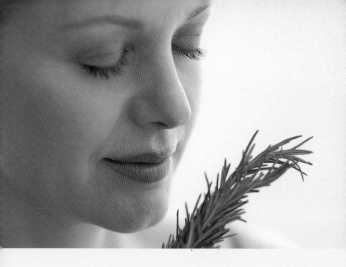
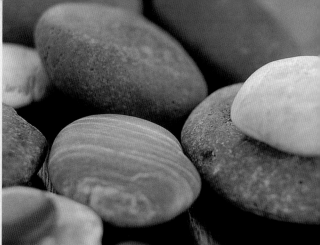

the whole body and require intense mental focus. A sequence of tai chi movements is called a form, and if you practice these forms on a regular basis, they'll help you stay physically healthy, mentally sharp, and spiritually grounded. Some forms are difficult; the exercises we've included are simple enough for anyone to try at home.

general fitness

A strong body gives you the foundation for moving with confidence through the world. People who are fit tend to feel more capable and energetic; they also reduce their risks of getting some diseases, of becoming obese, and of falling and suffering physical injuries. We've chosen a variety of general fitness exercises to help you strengthen your body and enliven your workout routine.

food and nutrition

Women in most countries have access to a greater variety of healthy foods—and more information on eating healthily—than ever before. Unfortunately, women also have access to a lot of unhealthy foods, unhealthy diet schemes, and media images of unhealthily thin models. That combination can make it hard to remember to eat the foods that most nourish our bodies and minds, even though research has confirmed that the foods we eat contribute to how we feel, what we weigh, and what diseases we get. You'll find carefully chosen (and tasty) recipes throughout this book, because we firmly believe that health (and happiness) come from what you put in your body, not just what you do with it.

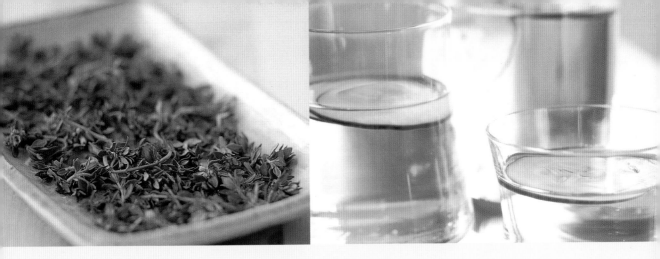

a few notes of caution

Some of the activities described in this book could be dangerous if performed incorrectly. When performing the physical exercises, for example, please take the time to read the text—don't just look at the pictures—and never push so hard that your body hurts. When you're practicing massage, it's important to remember not to massage directly on top of the spine or over varicose veins, open wounds, areas of intense pain, skin rashes, infections, or bruises. If you're pregnant, avoid exercises that impact the abdomen and those requiring deep work on your hands or feet. Pregnant women also shouldn't experiment with aromatherapy, and anyone using essential oils should read the instructions and warnings on the product labels before even opening the bottles. For instance, essential oils are almost never to be applied undiluted directly on the skin, and people with high blood pressure should avoid using stimulating oils. Finally, although the recipes we included in this book were designed for healthy eating, you should always take into account any dietary restrictions, such as limitations on sodium, or medical conditions, such as high cholesterol, that make a particular recipe inadvisable for you.

KEY TO THE ICONS

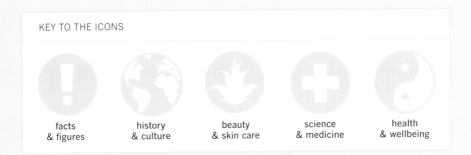

facts
& figures

history
& culture

beauty
& skin care

science
& medicine

health
& wellbeing

energize

Refreshed, renewed, and ready for anything. We all need a little help feeling energized from time to time, whether it's getting going first thing in the morning or recharging our batteries in the middle of a hectic day.

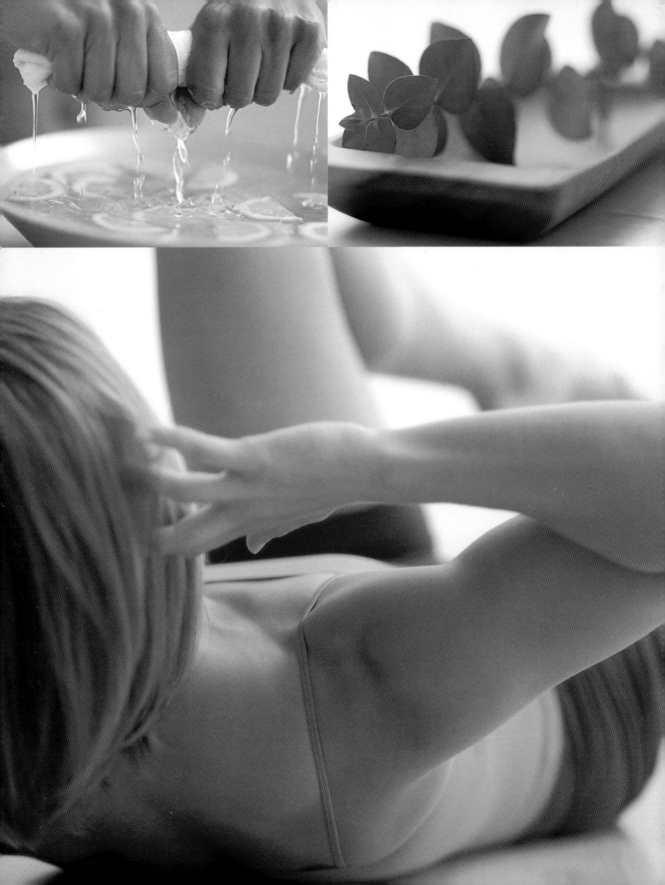

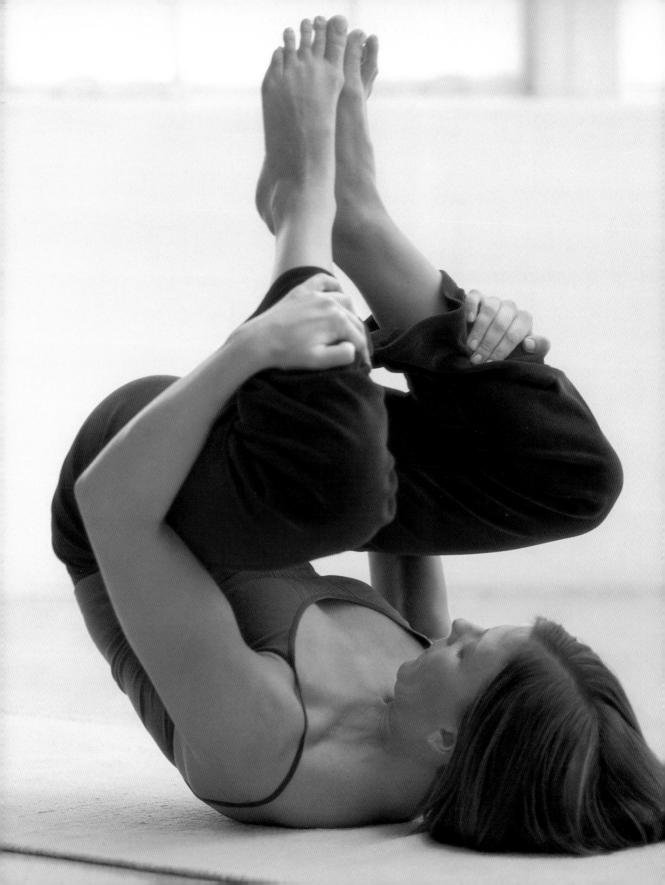

energize

With all the things we'd like to do—let alone have to do—it's no wonder that few of us are able to breeze through the day with energy to spare. In fact, chronic fatigue is one of the most common complaints doctors hear. Sometimes illness is to blame, but far more often the energy-sapping culprits are lifestyle factors such as poor diet, too little sleep, overscheduling, and, above all, stress.

If overscheduling is your nemesis, no one can wave a magic wand and add a few more hours to your 24/7 (wouldn't that be nice?). But you can rethink your work, family, and social commitments, and learn to say no to the ones that are less pleasurable or pressing. If a lack of sleep is your downfall, the solution is obvious—get more of it—but, in reality, that can be hard to do (see the Retreat chapter on page 174 ▶ for some tips). Taking a long, hard look at dietary habits is a good thing for everyone to do from time to time, and you'll find plenty of ideas for healthy eating in this book. If you're feeling stressed—the number one cause of chronic fatigue—the exercises, treatments, and activities in this chapter are guaranteed to help you handle everyday stress better and put a little more zip in your step.

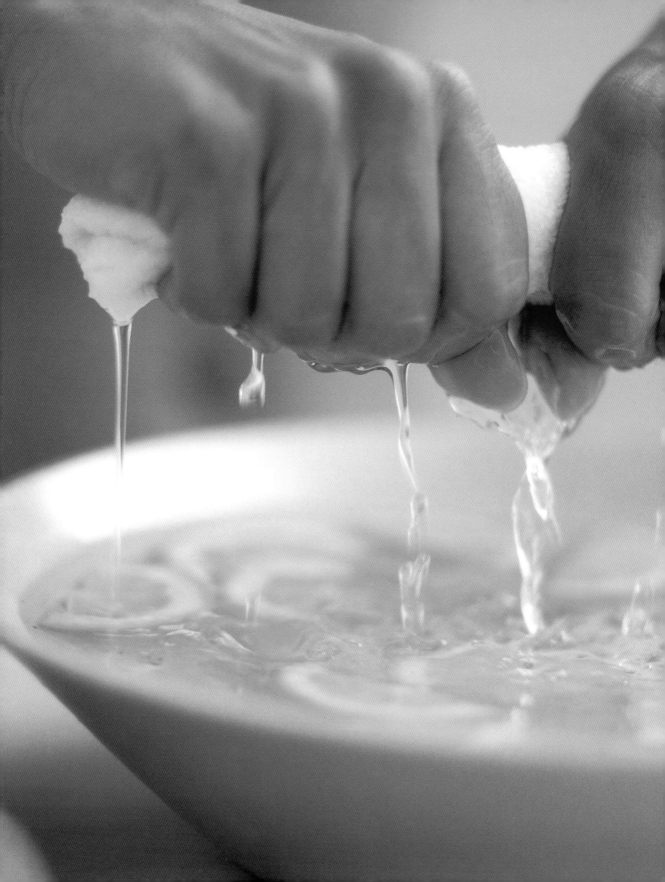

lemon scrub

Aromatherapists say that lemon, with its fresh and bracing scent, is one of the most beneficial essential oils for stimulating the mind and increasing alertness.

Start off your day with this refreshing treatment or simply try it as a pick-me-up before going out on the town: Add lemon essential oil and fresh lemon slices to a small bowl of warm water (see recipe at right). Place a clean washcloth in the bowl to soak, allowing it to become infused with lemon oil. After a couple minutes, swipe the cloth over any remaining oil droplets floating on top of the water, then wring it out. Place the cloth within easy reach of your shower.

Run a warm shower (if you make it too hot, it will make you feel listless, not invigorated). Briefly cleanse your body, using a citrus-scented soap if possible, and rinse off thoroughly. After turning off the shower, fold the washcloth into a compact square and begin scrubbing your body with it. Start at your feet and move upward, always scrubbing toward your heart, which helps stimulate your circulatory system. Towel off, and keep that fresh feeling going by applying a citrus-scented body moisturizer.

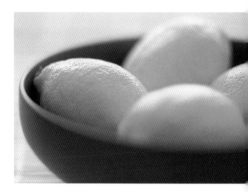

Fresh Lemon Scrub

5 drops lemon essential oil

6 or more fresh lemon slices

Small bowl of warm water

Washcloth

Citrus-scented soap (optional)

Citrus-scented body moisturizer

A LONG AND FRUITFUL HISTORY

Lemons are believed to have first been cultivated in the Indus Valley around 2500 B.C. Since then, in large part thanks to Arab traders, lemons have been prized by many cultures: They have earned mention in both the oldest known Chinese literature and the plays of Aristophanes, a Greek playwright in the fifth century B.C. The Romans believed lemons were antidotes to even the strongest poison, and their likeness graces the mosaics of Pompeii. During the reign of Louis XIV, French noblewomen bit into lemons to impart a rosy hue to their lips, and 19th-century British sailors carried them on board to ward off scurvy, often mixing the sour juice with a liberal helping of rum.

Lemony Skin-Care Benefits

Lemons contain generous amounts of vitamin C, a powerful antioxidant, as well as healthy helpings of citric acid and vitamins A and B_1. These helpful components are thought to encourage the exfoliation of dead skin, stimulate circulation, balance overactive oil glands, soften wrinkles, and help brighten the complexion. In a pinch, lemon juice diluted with water makes an effective toner.

tai chi opening sequence

This exercise encourages the flow of energy throughout the body. Usually done at the start of a tai chi session, it can be practiced on its own for a stimulating effect.

Not-So-Slow Going

Sure, tai chi is performed at a leisurely pace and the movements seem simple, making it appear far from an energizing experience. But take another look. Even though those gentle, flowing motions are done oh-so-slowly, they still get your heart pumping, your limbs loosened, your mind engaged, and your whole body working. Also, as a form of moving meditation, tai chi is extremely helpful in relieving stress, the most potent energy zapper out there.

1 With your eyes closed, spine straight, and feet close together, begin to clear your mind of thoughts and worries. Concentrate on the idea of gathering *chi* (or energy) in your body (see page 244 ▶). Breathe deeply and naturally. Spend a minute or two just quieting your mind and concentrating on awakening your dormant energy.

2 Open your eyes and step out to the side with one foot so your feet are shoulder-width apart; let your arms simply hang loosely at your sides. Imagine your weight settling down toward the earth.

3 Leading with your wrists, float your arms up to shoulder height, with the elbows and wrists slightly bent, palms facing in and fingers pointing down. Throughout the sequence, remember to keep your shoulders dropped and relaxed. Your legs should also be relaxed and still. Tuck in your tailbone (you do not want your buttocks to stick out) and keep your chin slightly down.

4 Now move down into a shallow squat—make sure that your knees always stay softly bent, with your toes pointed forward and the knees positioned directly above your toes. As you begin to squat, lead with your wrists and allow your elbows to sink and your forearms to float up, with your fingers pointing up and your palms facing out. As you rise, let your elbows flow up again and let your hands drop back down. Repeat the up-and-down motions eight times. While you work, think about maintaining good mental and physical form as you flow up and down: In tai chi, the aim is to keep the body relaxed, the joint angles soft, and the mind focused.

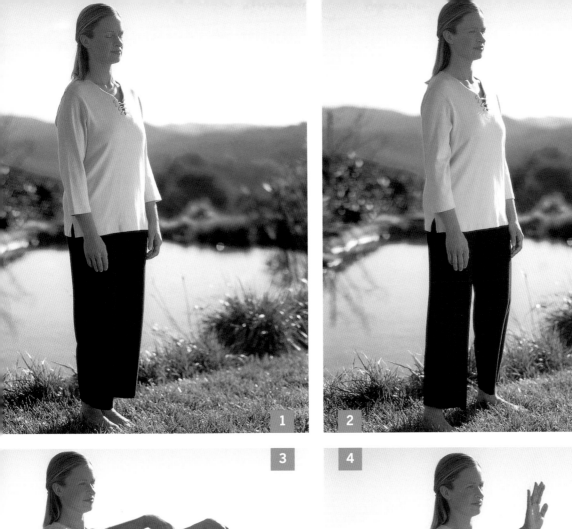

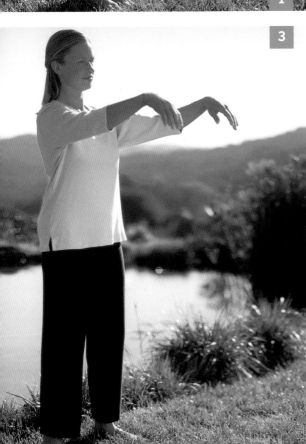

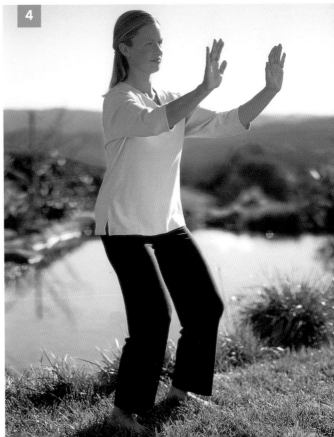

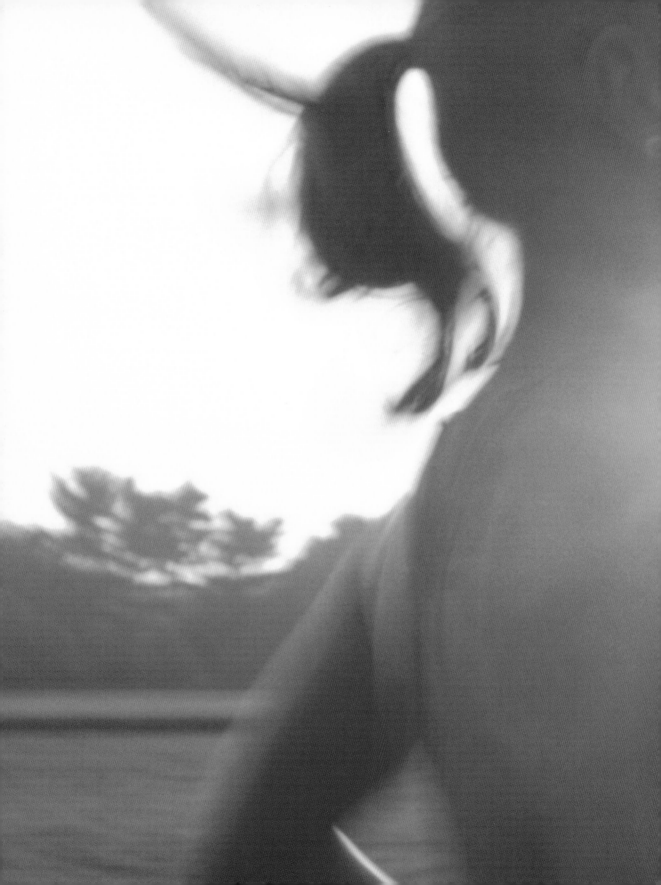

Yes, the gym's well equipped with the latest weight machines and you can easily keep up in your step-aerobics class. Pedaling your stationary bike lets you slip in a little exercise while you peruse the morning paper, and you feel the burn when you run through your buff-your-bum-for-beginners videotape. But nothing revitalizes a tired exercise routine or provides a treat for mind and body like getting into the great outdoors for a vigorous workout.

go outside and play

The options are myriad, and, with a little experimentation, you're sure to find the right ones for you. Maybe it's mountain biking or in-line skating. Maybe it's hiking nearby trails or swimming laps in a local pool. Take your tai chi routine to a park, or sign up for those kayaking lessons you've always talked about. Make the most of the season, and go skiing or snowboarding, run on the beach, or ride a horse through an autumnal forest. (Don't let chilly weather serve as an excuse to keep you house- or gym-bound; you actually burn around 5 percent more calories when you exercise in the cold, because your body has to work harder to maintain its core temperature—more bang for your exercise buck.) No matter what form of outdoor activity you choose, you're sure to find that fresh air and fresh scenery result in a fresh attitude. There's an added bonus, too: Changing your exercise habits (see page 309 ▶) will allow you to work out new parts of your mind and body.

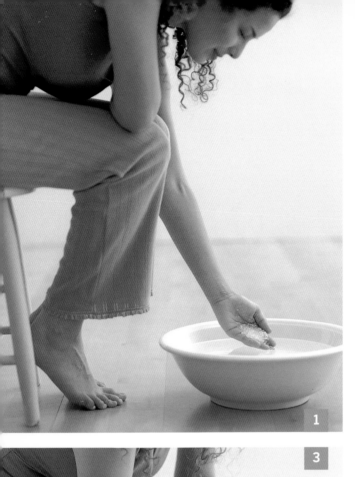

1

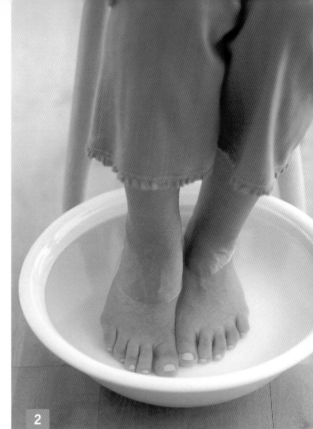

2

3

4

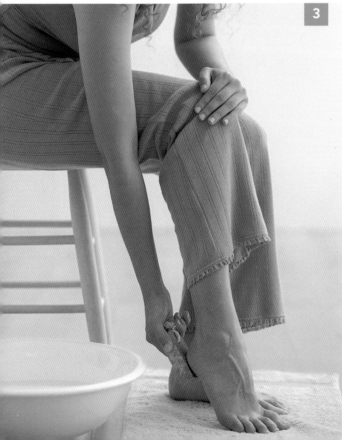

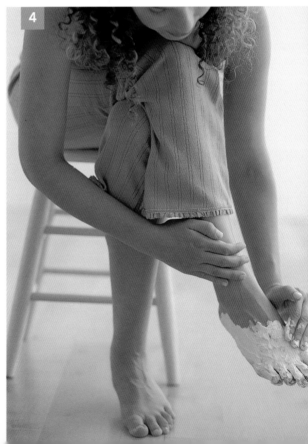

peppermint foot spa

Powered by one of the most versatile and refreshing aromatic oils, this invigorating foot treatment is a sure bet for putting a new bounce in your step.

1 Fill a large bowl with warm water, making sure that the water level will fall just below your ankles. Add one heaping tablespoon of peppermint oil mineral crystals to the water.

2 Soak your feet for at least ten minutes to soften and refresh your skin. Aside from being immensely soothing, the foot bath will make the next step—exfoliation—easier and more effective.

3 After thoroughly drying your feet, use a pumice stone to smooth out any rough patches on your heels. Firmly rub the stone up and down from the back of your heel to the bottom of your foot. Continue until the skin feels smoother. Repeat on the other foot.

4 If you have a little more time, follow up with a hydrating and energizing foot mask. Spread a thick layer of the mask over the tops and soles of your feet and in between your toes. Apply gently, and don't rub in. Leave on for 15 minutes, then thoroughly remove the mask by wiping with a wet washcloth or rinsing in the bathtub.

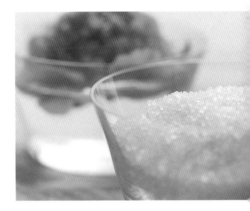

The Power of Peppermint
Peppermint has been used for everything from relieving headaches to soothing upset stomachs. This popular medicinal plant is credited with being a nasal decongestant and a powerful mental stimulant. Its prime active component is menthol. When applied to the skin, menthol quickly produces a cooling sensation, which the body reacts to by increasing blood flow to the area, creating a comforting sense of warmth.

FEET, DON'T FAIL ME NOW

Ever notice that when your feet feel tired your whole energy level takes a downturn? It's no wonder, when you consider the demands we place on our poor feet, intricate structures consisting of 26 bones, 30 finely tuned muscles, and 114 ligaments. On average, human feet take a pounding of 10,000 steps daily, with each of those steps subjecting these relatively small structures to about three times our weight. For runners, the feet are more susceptible to injury than any other part, with heel pain caused by inflammation the most frequent complaint. In general, though, corns are the most common foot problem.

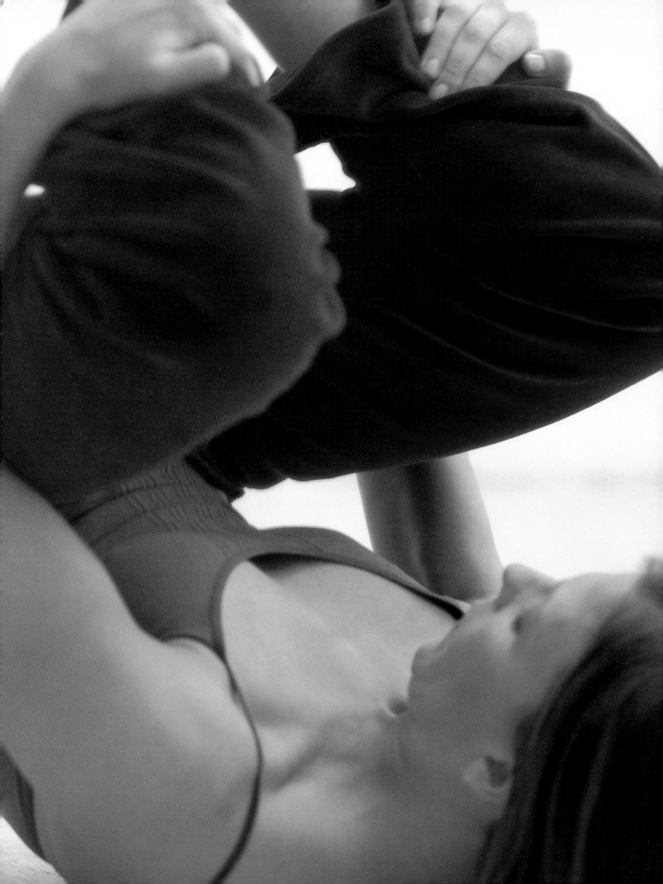

morning energizer

Skip the caffeine and start your day with a Pilates workout to clarify your mind and loosen your body, making you focused, flexible, and ready to go.

Sure, you can turn to lattes and chocolate croissants for a rush of morning energy. But the highs you get from caffeine and sugar can first make you jittery and then leave you tired—plus the substances themselves aren't great for your body. You can develop more sustained energy by practicing Pilates, a system of slow, focused exercises that are designed to elongate the body, increase flexibility, strengthen muscles, and focus the mind. Variations of these exercises, based on the original work of Joseph Pilates (a German who deeply believed in the importance of mental and physical conditioning), are now taught in fitness studios around the world.

The benefits of a morning Pilates routine, such as the one outlined on the next page, are obvious. Strong muscles moving freely (that is, not bound by pain or stiffness) naturally impart more energy. And a calm mind (one not jangled by stress) naturally feels much clearer.

EXERCISING'S ENERGY BOOST

Studies have shown that exercising can fight fatigue and brighten your outlook. In one American study, researchers concluded that female college students who rode stationary bicycles at a moderate clip for as little as ten minutes a day showed "significant declines in levels of fatigue and confusion and significant improvements in energy levels." The fact that the participants got such results from relatively little exercise is especially good news for sedentary women reluctant to commit to a strenuous, time-consuming routine. Fitness researcher James Annesi, who has also studied exercise's psychological effects, says, "Meeting small goals can boost your energy and your self-esteem, keeping you motivated."

step-by-step sequence ▶

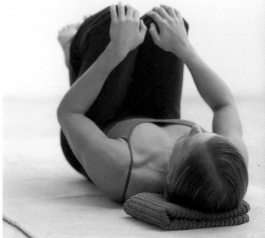

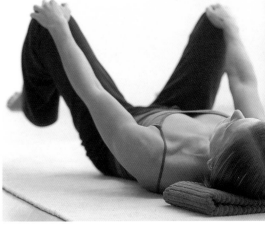

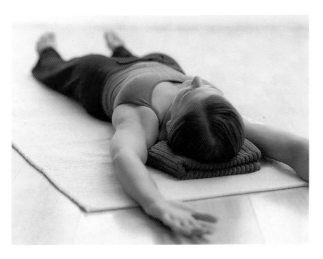

1 To begin, lie on your back on a mat or other comfortably padded surface; if you like, you can use a folded towel as a pillow to cushion your head. Keep your legs hip-width apart, your arms stretched out way overhead, and your fingers spread wide. Push through the balls of your feet so that you lengthen your spine, but don't arch your back.

2 Bend your knees, so your thighs are perpendicular to the floor while your lower legs dangle. Place your hands on top of your knees. Maintain a little space between the floor and the small of your back.

3 Lightly pressing your palms down on your knees, circle your legs away from each other, down away from the torso, and around back together. Keep your pelvis steady. Circle eight times, then eight times in the other direction.

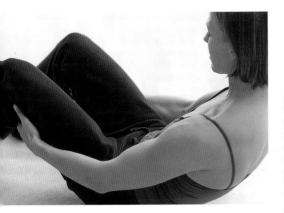

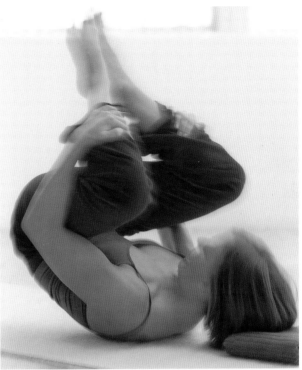

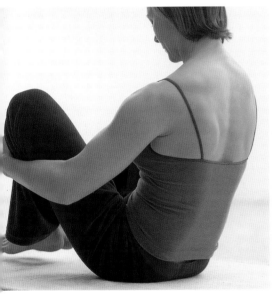

6 Tighten your abdominals, round your lower back, open your knees, and hold onto the front of your shins with your hands. Keep your elbows wide and your chin slightly tucked in. Staying rounded in a little ball, rock back and forth on your back. Avoid rocking onto your neck. Concentrate on inhaling as you rock backward and exhaling as you rock upward. Repeat eight times.

4 With your legs bent and your hands on the backs of your thighs, roll up using your abs. Slowly roll back down to the ground, rounding your back and pressing the back of your rib cage to the floor. Roll back up. Repeat eight times.

5 Roll up again and sit with your feet on or off the floor (use whichever position is easier for you). If they're off the floor, balance on your buttocks.

invigorating massage

Not all massages are meant to soothe. The brisk motions in this technique are perfect for revving up before a workout or a demanding day at work.

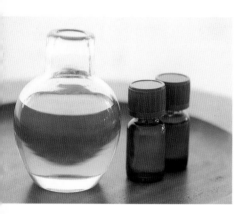

Energizing Massage Blend

2 ounces carrier oil (such as grape
    seed, jojoba, or sweet almond oil)
16 drops geranium essential oil
7 drops rosemary essential oil
2 drops peppermint essential oil

Keeping It Short and Sweet
Invigorating sports massages can be beneficial either before or after a workout. They are usually short in duration, with just a few minutes being restorative without being overly relaxing for the recipient. The brief rubdowns also give the hardworking massager a break, as they require quite a bit of energy to give.

Recruit a friend to give you this invigorating massage treatment, which is particularly ideal when you're under a lot of stress. Begin the massage lying facedown on a firm, comfortable surface, and ask your friend to follow these four steps:

1 Warm some massage oil (see the recipe at left) between your palms and spread a light, even layer across your friend's back and sides. Starting at the waist, press your hands up along each side of the spine, gliding to the top. Fan your hands out across her shoulders, swing your fingers down along the ribs and sides, and pull your hands back to the waist. Keep your hands and fingers relaxed and molded to the contours of the body. Apply more pressure as you stroke up, less as you stroke down. Continue for several minutes.

2 With your friend faceup or facedown, spread massage oil evenly onto one leg. Using gliding motions, encircle as much of her leg as possible. Lead the stroke with the web of your hand (the skin between the thumb and index finger). Start at the ankle and move over the calf and thigh using firm pressure (use light pressure on the knee); glide back toward the ankle with lighter pressure. Stroke slowly, then speed up for two minutes. Repeat on the other leg.

3 Lift one of her hands, and firmly glide your other hand from her wrist to elbow to arm socket; glide lightly back to the wrist. Lead the stroke with the web of your cupped hand. Establish a brisk pattern for about one minute. Repeat on the other arm.

4 Knead her back. Gently work smaller muscles with your thumb and fingertips in a motion like a cat's paw opening and closing in contentment. Push and pull larger muscles with wider, deeper movements, as if kneading dough. Continue for a few minutes.

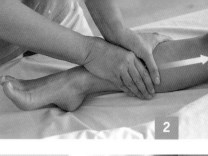

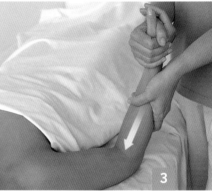

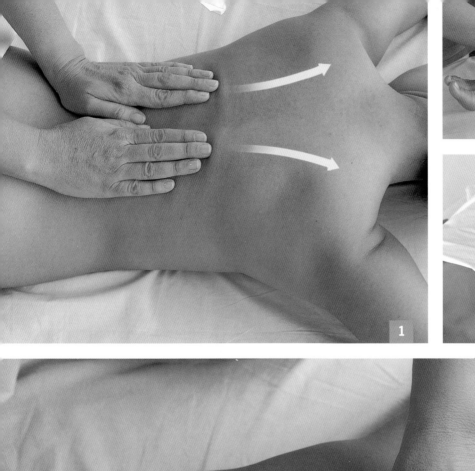

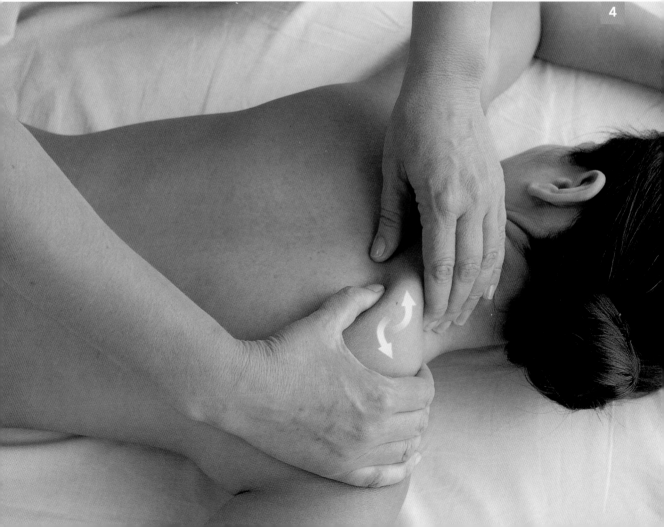

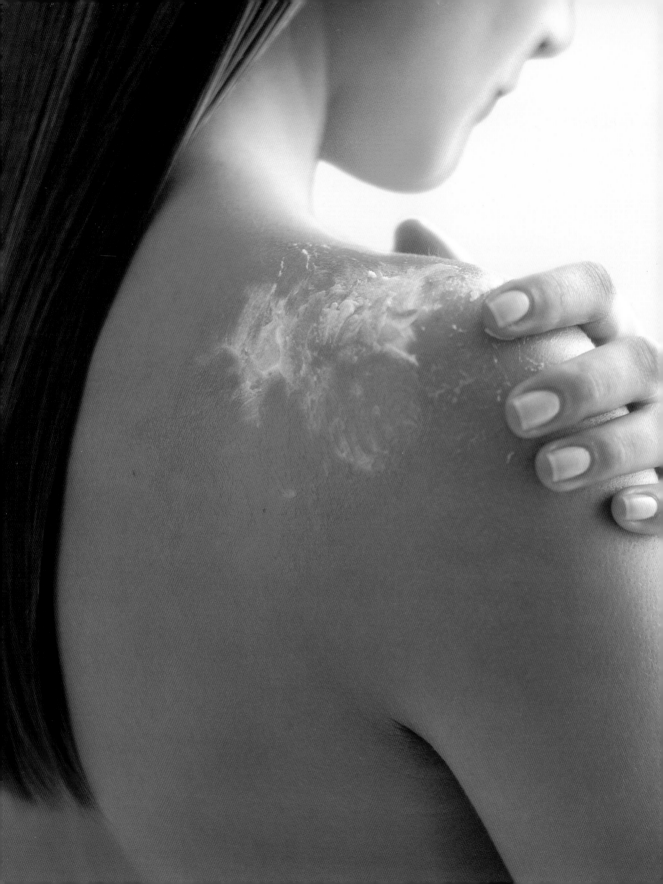

eucalyptus body lotion

After your shower, take time for a step that can make a big difference to the rest of your day: Moisturize, from top to toes, using a product with a refreshing scent.

Take a warm, brief shower and dry off lightly, leaving your skin slightly damp. This helps trap some of the moisture in your skin when you apply the body lotion. Starting with your shoulders and working downward, apply a liberal amount of moisturizer, rubbing it in well and putting a little extra on dry patches of skin.

The scent you choose can have a big effect on your mood, and if it's energy you're craving, eucalyptus (pictured at right) simply can't be beat. Its bracing aroma is a wake-up call for the mind; its chemical components act as both a deodorant and stimulant for the body. If the scent doesn't appeal to you, explore other energizing essential oils such as rosemary, cypress, bay laurel, and basil. Lemon and orange are also refreshing, but be aware that they heighten photosensitivity.

You can use a preformulated product or just add a few drops of eucalyptus essential oil—or a blend of oils (see recipe at right)—to an unscented moisturizer. You're not limited to lotion here; there are many different types of moisturizers. If your skin is very dry, a scented oil, a body butter, or a cream moisturizer will leave it feeling soft and well hydrated. If your skin is normal, either a cream or an emollient-rich body lotion probably will do the trick. If your skin is oily or prone to pimples, stick to a lighter body lotion, making sure that it's non-comedogenic (which means that it won't clog pores).

You'll find hundreds of choices in each category, so you may need to experiment to find the one that has just the right scent and feel for you. Take advantage of testers in stores, and keep in mind that products that seem overly greasy, sticky, or thick in the jar or tube might melt wonderfully into your skin once applied. Also notice which ones have staying power; some will keep your thirsty skin feeling hydrated much longer than others.

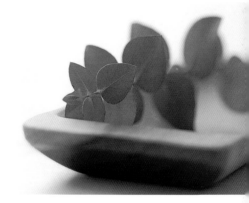

Bracing Body Lotion

2 ounces unscented lotion

10 drops eucalyptus essential oil

7 drops rosemary essential oil

5 drops pine essential oil

3 drops lemongrass essential oil

Fragrant Remedies
Indigenous to Australia and its neighboring islands, the eucalyptus tree has been a source of spiritual and medicinal remedies for centuries. Today, fragrant eucalyptus oil is in countless products, helping to relieve stuffed-up noses, soothe sore throats, kill germs, improve blemished skin, and alleviate muscle aches.

hand reflexology

Human bodies have zones of energy, according to reflexologists, who recommend activating these zones to improve health and enhance feelings of wellbeing.

Reflexology is the practice of applying firm pressure to specific points on the hands and feet to exert influence on other body parts, organs, glands, and systems. The theory is that these reflexology points are linked by neurological and energy pathways to specific and often far-removed parts of the body. Pressure on a given point is thought to clear any energy blockages and to have either a stimulating or relaxing effect. All you need is a reflexology map (see the illustration at left) to guide you to the pertinent points on your hands (also see page 201 ► for a sample reflexology map of the feet).

1 To awaken your internal organs in the morning, stimulate their reflexology points by pressing the thumb of one of your hands deeply into the palm of your other hand. Move your thumb in little circles from the bottom of the palm to the base of each finger. (Another method is to position your thumb in the center of the palm and rock the palm onto the tip of your thumb. Then rock the palm off the thumb, move your thumb to a new position, and repeat the sequence.) Make sure that you cover the palm's entire surface. Keep in mind that steady, direct pressure is used to help reduce pain, while pressing and releasing (often called alternating pressure) helps stimulate the point. When you identify a body part that seems to warrant particular attention, try working its corresponding reflexology point for at least 30 seconds.

2 To stimulate energy in the reflexology zones in your sinuses, head, brain, neck, and throat, firmly press and circle the tip of each finger and the length of the thumb. Work both hands.

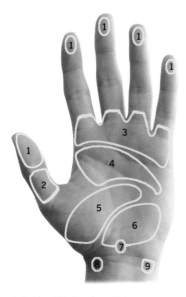

Left Hand Reflexology Points
Here are some of the key reflexology points on the palm side of your left hand:

1 Sinus, head, and brain
2 Neck and throat
3 Eye and ear
4 Lung, breast, back, and heart
5 Stomach and pancreas
6 Intestines
7 Bladder
8 Uterus
9 Ovary

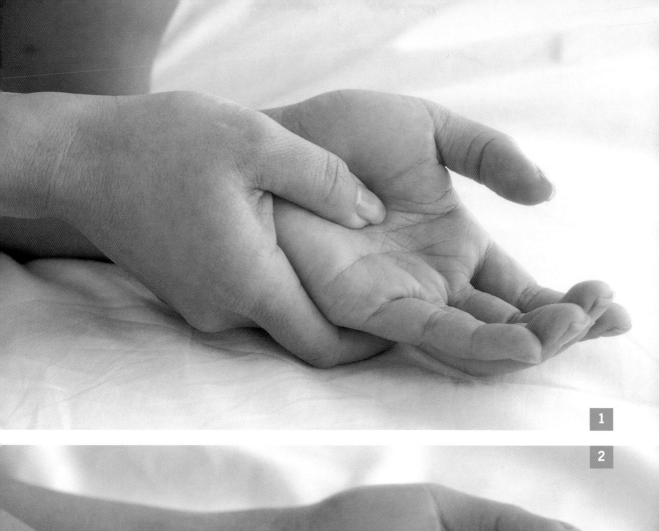

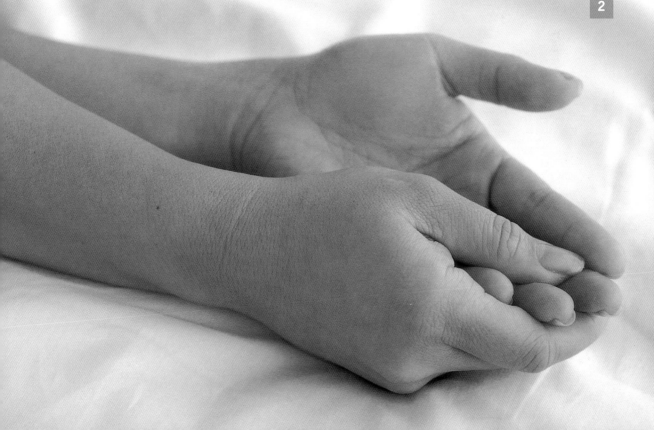

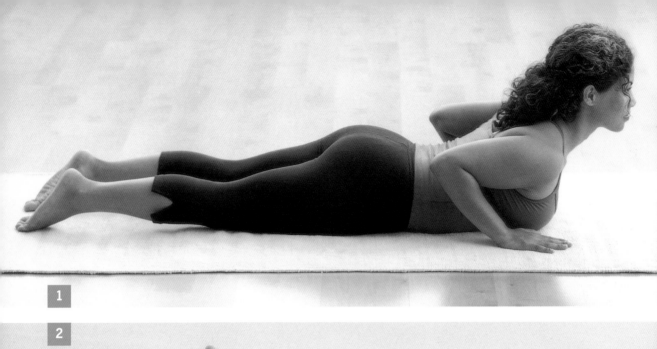

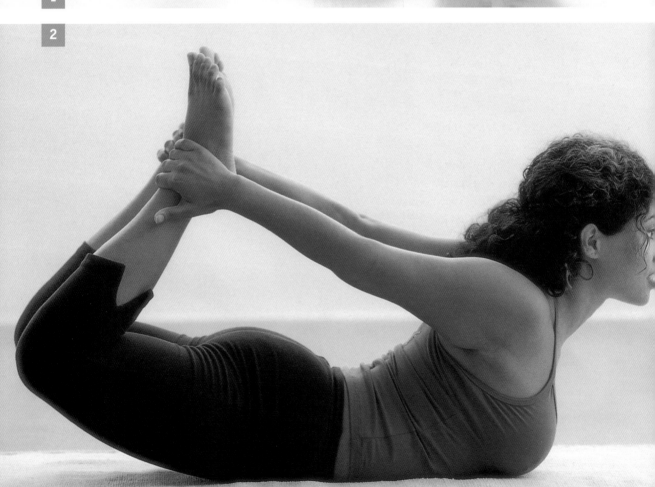

cobra and bow

Backward-bending yoga poses build strength, exert gentle pressure on the adrenal glands, and allow you to breathe more deeply, bestowing a sense of vigor.

1 To perform the Cobra pose (also known as an *asana*), lie facedown on a comfortable surface. Set your feet hip-width apart and point your toes. Resting your forehead on the floor, place your palms flat on the floor directly beneath your shoulders, bringing your elbows in toward your ribs. Inhale and gently extend your chin forward as you lift your head, neck, and chest as high as you can comfortably without putting pressure on your palms. Keep your shoulder blades low. Hold the pose for four to ten breaths, then release.

2 The Bow pose is more challenging. Still facedown on the floor, bend your knees and bring your heels toward your hips; reach back to grasp your feet or ankles, whichever position is more comfortable. Allow your legs to separate, but keep your heels over your buttocks. Inhale, and raise your head, neck, chest, and thighs, pressing your feet into your hands and lifting your heels away from your back. The quality of your effort is more important than how far your legs or chest lift up, so don't strain. Hold for four to six breaths. While exhaling the last time, slowly lower yourself back down to the floor.

A Muscular Balancing Act
Your back muscles stabilize your spinal column, allowing you to stand upright and bend and straighten your body. They provide support for your chest and extra power for your arms. These muscles also work in concert with your abdominal muscles to assist in breathing and protect your internal organs. Maintaining a balance between the two muscle groups is vital, so it's wise to pair back-strengthening poses like these with abdominal exercises such as the ones found on page 81 ▶.

ENERGIZING YOGA TIPS

To feel more energized in the morning, Ayurvedic yogis recommend a variety of practices that go far beyond starting the day with a yoga routine. They involve everything from the hour you rise to the foods you eat for breakfast. Ayurveda, the traditional medicine of India, is a centuries-old holistic health-care system. In Sanskrit, *ayur* means "life" and *veda* means "knowledge." The system teaches how to balance our life energies and achieve harmony with the environment, returning us to a natural state of health and happiness.

AYURVEDIC EYE-OPENERS

- Rise at least 20 minutes before the sun does.
- Splash cool water on your face seven times.
- Drink a glass of lukewarm water garnished with a lemon or lime slice.
- Use a tongue scraper, gently moving it from the back of the tongue to the front.
- Tap your teeth together to stimulate the *nadis*, channels through which energy flows.

energize

curried eggs on bread

This satisfying anytime dish combines the complex carbohydrates of whole grains with the high-quality protein of eggs to give you energy to burn.

Ingredients

6 hard-boiled eggs

⅓ cup low-fat mayonnaise, or to taste

1 tablespoon Dijon mustard

½ teaspoon curry powder

½ teaspoon Tabasco green jalapeño
sauce

Kosher salt and freshly ground pepper

1 to 2 tablespoons minced fresh chives

4 slices of whole-grain bread

• Serves: 4

• Prep time: 10 minutes

• Cook time: 10–15 minutes (for
hard-boiled eggs)

With all the hype surrounding low-carb diets, it's easy to forget that carbohydrates are the body's main source of energy. But some carbs are superior nutritionally to others, and they should be incorporated into a balanced diet. Here's an easy recipe that gives you plenty of protein and complex carbohydrates—perfect fuel to rev you up and keep you going. (Note: Most nutritionists now say that, unless you have high blood cholesterol levels, you can eat five egg yolks a week.)

1 Peel and coarsely chop the eggs. Place in a medium-size bowl.

2 In a small bowl, combine the mayonnaise, mustard, curry powder, and jalapeño sauce. Pour the mixture onto the eggs and stir to combine. Add salt and pepper to taste. Fold in the chopped chives.

3 Spread on the bread slices to make open-faced sandwiches.

Nutritional Information Per Serving

Whole-grain breads, such as whole wheat, give this meal its energy boost.

Calories	220
Kilojoules	940
Protein	12 g
Carbohydrates	19 g
Total Fat	10 g
Saturated Fat	2.5 g
Cholesterol	320 mg
Sodium	530 mg
Dietary Fiber	2 g

NOT ALL CARBS ARE CREATED EQUAL

Even the diet books that urge people to cut back (sometimes way back) on their consumption of carbohydrates usually distinguish between good and bad carbs. Bad carbs include sugar and starchy foods such as potatoes, pasta, and foods made with white flour. These carbohydrates don't provide enough nutritional benefits to offset the fact that the body quickly converts them to sugar, later causing a slump in energy. Good carbs include fruits, vegetables, and the complex carbohydrates found in whole grains, legumes, and nuts. These take longer to convert to sugar and are rich in vitamins, minerals, fiber, antioxidants, and other key nutrients. Although hotly debated, the general recommendation from nutritional authorities is that at least half our calories should come from carbohydrates.

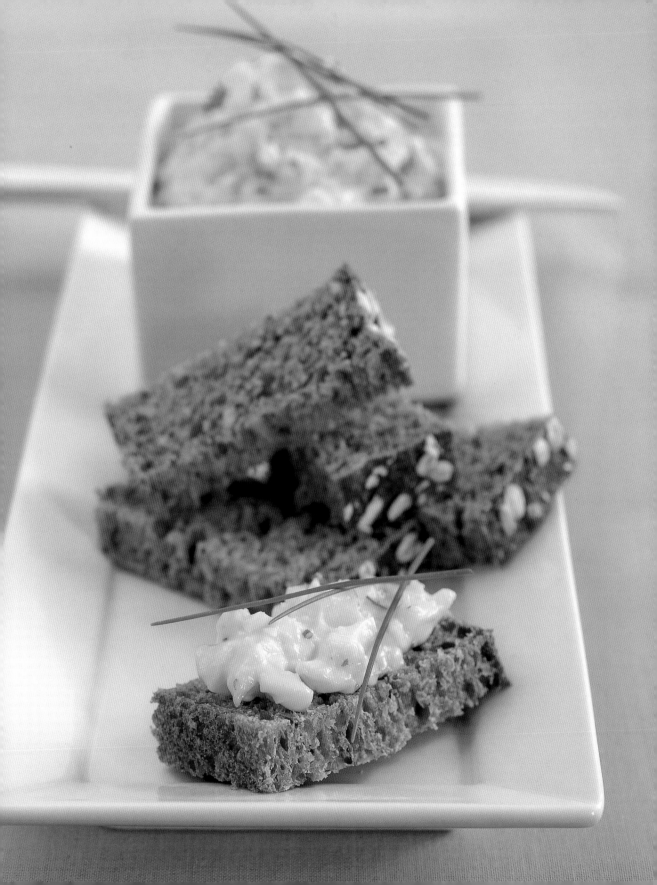

cleanse

Much more than a matter of good grooming and diligent hygiene, effective cleansing involves refreshing the mind and spirit as well as the body.

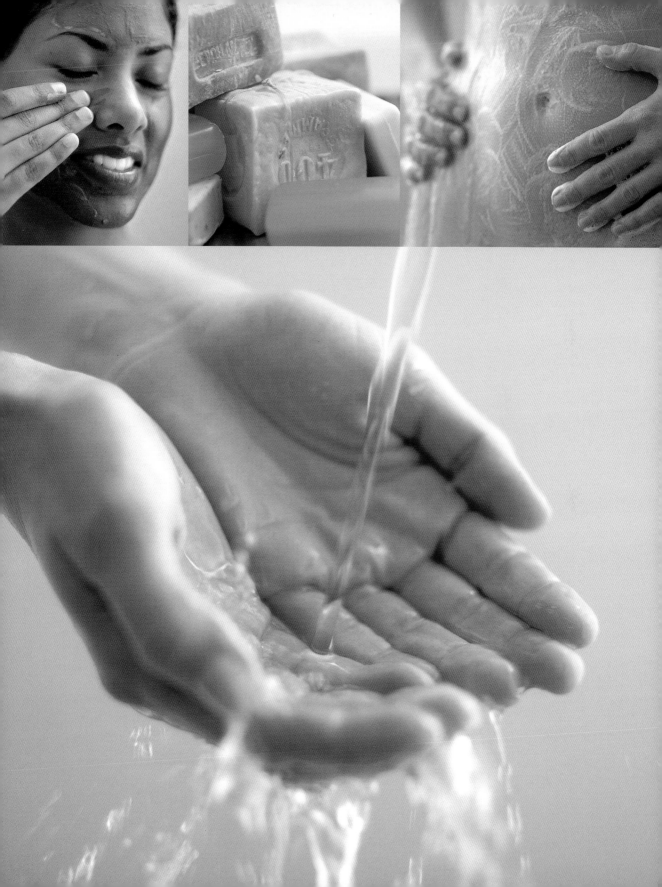

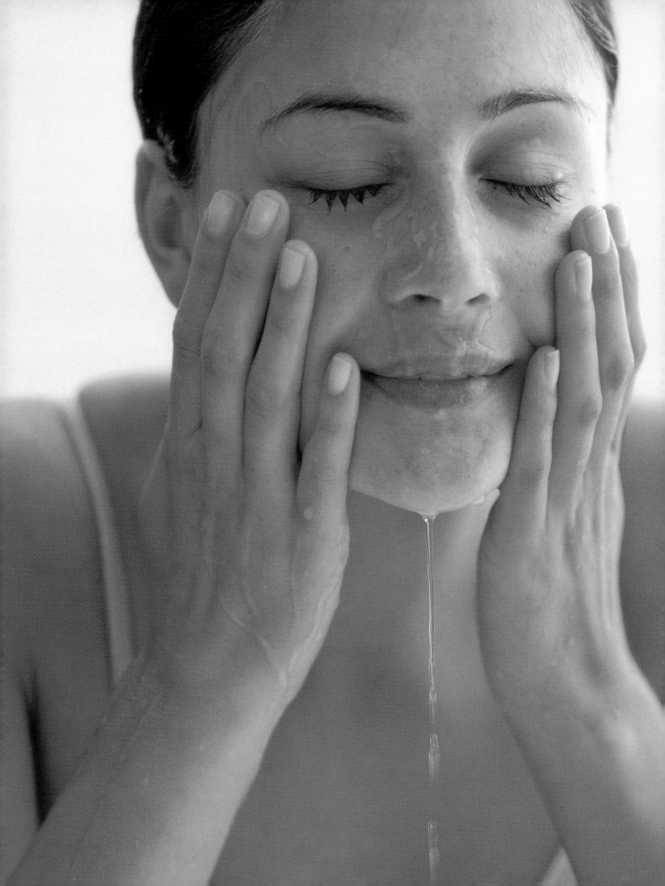

cleanse

When you contemplate the notion of cleansing, you are likely to think of mundane tasks such as washing your face and taking a shower. This chapter offers plenty of good advice on those essential daily rituals—as well as many other aspects of personal grooming—but it takes more than that to truly come clean.

Cleansing also involves sweeping away mental cobwebs of worry and negative thoughts, and purifying the spirit as well. What's more, as far as the body is concerned, there's the inside as well as the outside of our corporeal selves to consider. Cleansing means undoing some of the damage that poor nutrition, a lack of adequate exercise, and other bad habits—not to mention stress and environmental pollution—might have wreaked on our beleaguered bodies. This process might sound involved, and maybe even a little lofty, but on the following pages you'll find a wide variety of down-to-earth, accessible ideas for cleaning up your act.

identifying skin types

The first step in good skin care is determining your skin type: dry, oily, normal, or a combination. Then move on to mastering a few everyday-care essentials.

Your Skin's Changing Needs
Keep in mind that your skin type may change over time or because of factors such as diet, weather, hormones, and medications. Stay attuned to the way your skin is responding, and be ready to tweak your daily regimen when necessary.

Cosmetologists and skin-care specialists base their recommendations for cleansing, toning, and moisturing facial skin (see page 57 ▶) according to its degree of oiliness. Dry skin is usually oil starved, for example, and tends to be dull, rough, flaky, and fragile. The pores usually are small, and the skin often wrinkles prematurely.

Oily skin develops shiny patches a few hours after washing because of its overly enthusiastic oil production or an overabundance of oil glands. It often has a coarse texture, large pores, and a tendency to develop pimples and blackheads. The good news is that oily skin tends to be a bit more resistant to wrinkles.

Normal skin produces just enough oil to protect the uppermost layer and keep it supple without interfering with the natural process of shedding dead cells. It won't feel taut after being washed with a mild cleanser and water. The pores typically are medium size. In combination skin, the T-zone (the forehead, nose, and chin) is oily, while the areas around the eyes, cheeks, and neck may be dry

PHOTOSENSITIVITY SKIN TYPE	NO.
Always burns, never tans	I
Burns easily, tans slightly	II
Burns first, then usually tans evenly	III
Burns minimally, tans well	IV
Rarely burns, always develops deep tan	V
Almost never burns, may darken slightly	VI

FOLLOWING THE SUN

Dermatologists usually think of skin types in terms of sun sensitivity. Knowing your own level of UV sensitivity is important, as it can help you understand the precautions you should take to help reduce the chance of skin cancer and premature aging. If you're Type I, II, or III, be very diligent about using a sunscreen with an SPF (sun protection factor) of 15 or more. But don't get a false sense of security if you have a higher skin type: Even ebony skin offers a natural SPF of only 6 to 8. (See page 167 ▶ for information on self-tanning.)

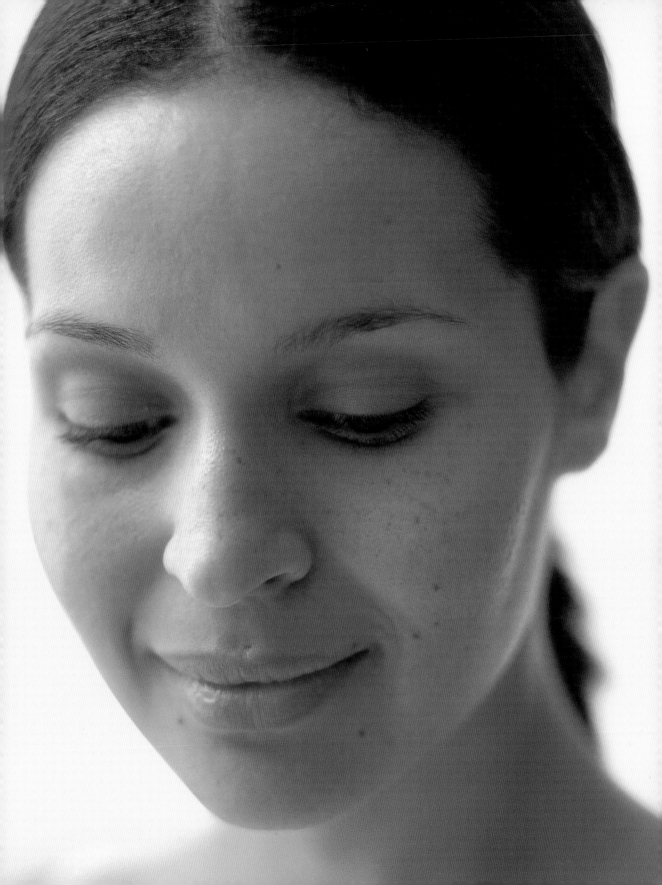

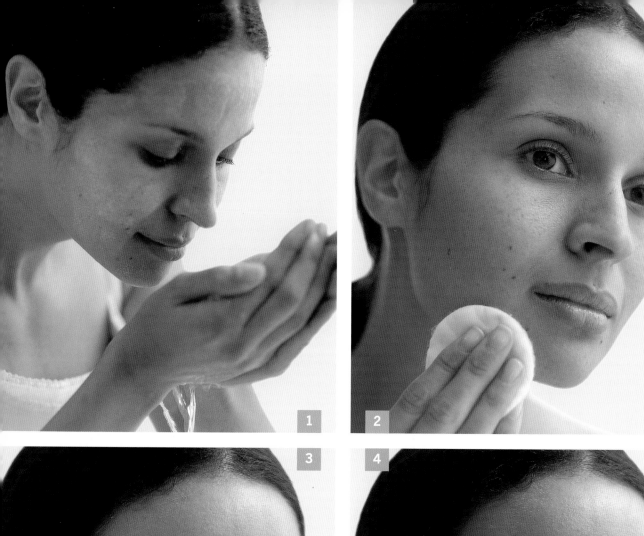

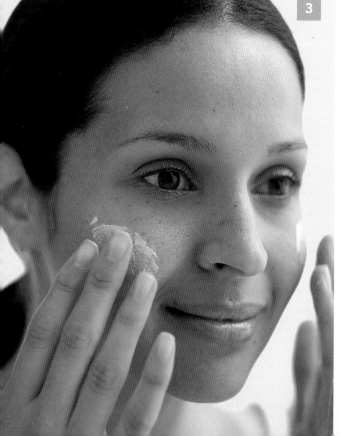

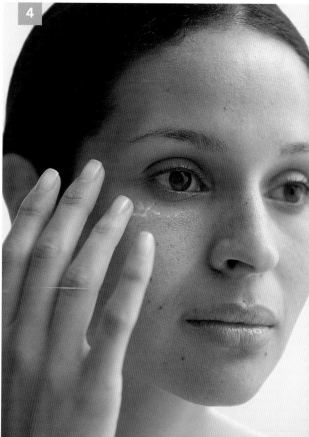

skin-care basics

Four basic steps—cleansing, toning, moisturizing, and caring for the eye area—will help you keep your facial skin looking and feeling its best.

1 Wash your face (twice a day is best, but at least every night!) with a cleanser formulated for your skin type (see page 54 ◄). Dry skin benefits from a cleansing milk or cream. Some product directions recommend simply wiping away the cleanser with a washcloth or tissue after massaging it in, but if your skin still feels a bit greasy, you can rinse off the cleanser with tepid water instead. If your skin is oily, it usually will respond well to a refreshing foam or gel. Normal skin can tolerate many forms of cleansing products, and which type you settle on is a matter of personal preference. (If you use a foam or bar-soap cleanser and your skin feels tight and dry shortly after washing, try switching to a slightly more emollient product.) For combination skin, you probably will need to cater to the oilier areas of your face by using a gel or foam cleanser, and then take care to moisturize properly (see Step 3).

2 Apply a toner, putting a small amount on a cotton pad and gently running it over your entire face. Toners or astringents help remove residual traces of make-up and impurities. Some cool and refresh (good for oily skin); some hydrate and soften (a plus for dry skin). For normal and combination skin, try a few types to see what works for you.

3 After the toner dries, apply moisturizer. An oil-free formula is best for oily skin, a richly emollient product nourishes dry skin, and something in between suits normal skin. If you have combination skin, apply an oil-free moisturizer to your T-zone (the forehead, nose, and chin) and a richer product to drier areas.

4 Take special care of the skin around your eyes, which is delicate and prone to wrinkles. Use a gentle eye-make-up remover every evening, plus an eye cream or gel morning and night. Pat it lightly under your eyes and at the outside corners (where crow's-feet form) with your ring finger, which is the weakest finger and the least likely to tug your skin.

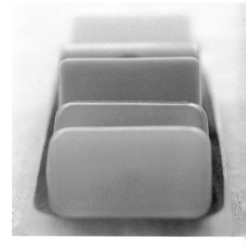

How Soap Works

Soaps break the rule that water and oil don't mix. A component of soap called *surfactant* has a molecular structure that attracts water on one end and non-water-soluble substances on the other. When you lather up, surfactant links oil (and dirt) to water; simply rinse and off come the dirt and oil adhered to it. A soap that is too harsh for your skin may have too much surfactant. Try a milder option.

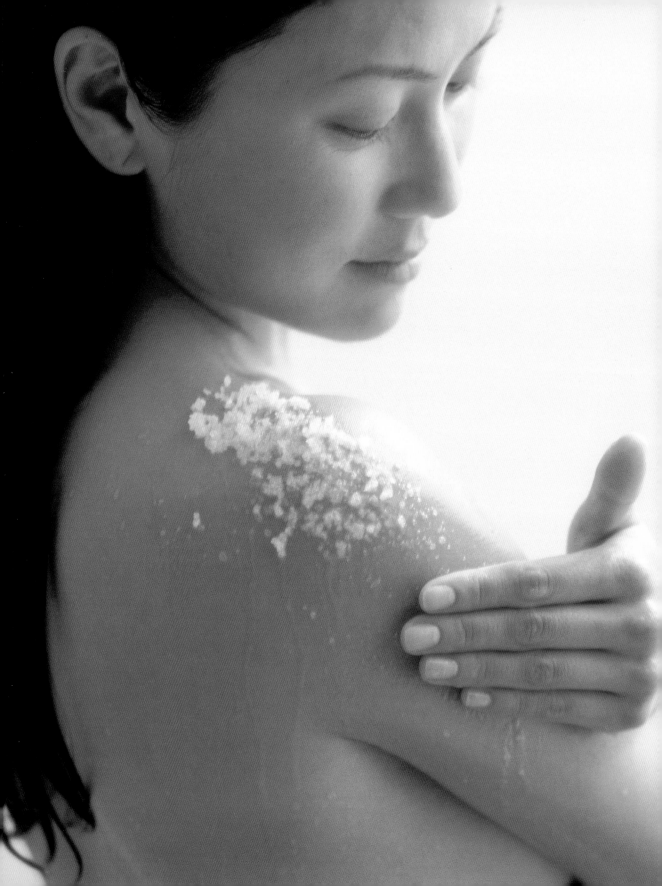

body exfoliation

An often neglected step in cleansing, manual exfoliation helps the body shed dead skin cells, exposing the healthier-looking, more radiant skin waiting just beneath.

As you shower or bathe, spread a small amount of cleansing gel on a sisal washcloth or mitt, or on a loofah, which is made from a vine-grown vegetable with a fleshy, fibrous interior. Work the gel into a lather and then rub the cloth or loofah all over your body, scrubbing toward your heart to aid the flow of lymphatic fluids.

You can achieve the same effect by skipping the rough-textured applicator and using an exfoliating scrub. First, cleanse as usual in the shower. After rinsing off all the soap or shower gel, turn off the shower. Using a preformulated sugar, sea salt, or nut scrub (or the recipe at right), scoop out about two tablespoons into your hand and apply the scrub firmly over your skin in small circular motions, starting with your feet and legs, then your arms. Pay special attention to any patches of dry skin, such as those often found on heels and elbows. Next, exfoliate your buttocks, stomach, back (well, as much as you can reach), and chest, decreasing pressure when working on delicate areas and adding more product as needed. Rinse with plenty of warm water, using your hands to help remove all the scrub.

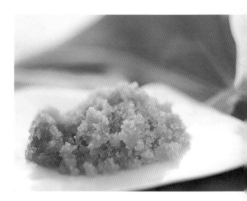

Sweet and Spicy Body Polish

1 tablespoon Demerara sugar

1 tablespoon golden brown sugar

1 tablespoon superfine sugar

4 tablespoons honey

2 teaspoons lemon or lime juice

1 teaspoon ground ginger

½ teaspoon ground cinnamon

GOING FOR THE GLOW

The body sheds up to 500 million dead cells daily from its upper layer, the epidermis. If these cells remained, they would form a thick layer, locking out moisture and making the skin appear dull or flaky. Manual exfoliation helps the body slough off dead cells, revealing a new layer of rosier skin. It also helps stimulate circulation, loosen ingrown hairs, and lift away dirt and excess oil. As we age, dead cells take longer to rise to the top of the epidermis and then slough off, so exfoliation becomes an increasingly important self-care ritual.

Too Much of a Good Thing

If your skin is dry or sensitive, don't use an exfoliating scrub *and* a sisal washcloth or loofah—that combination is likely to cause irritation. Also, never exfoliate sunburned or broken skin. Be sure to slather on a moisturizer (see page 43 ◂) after exfoliating, since the procedure can deplete the skin's reservoir of moisture.

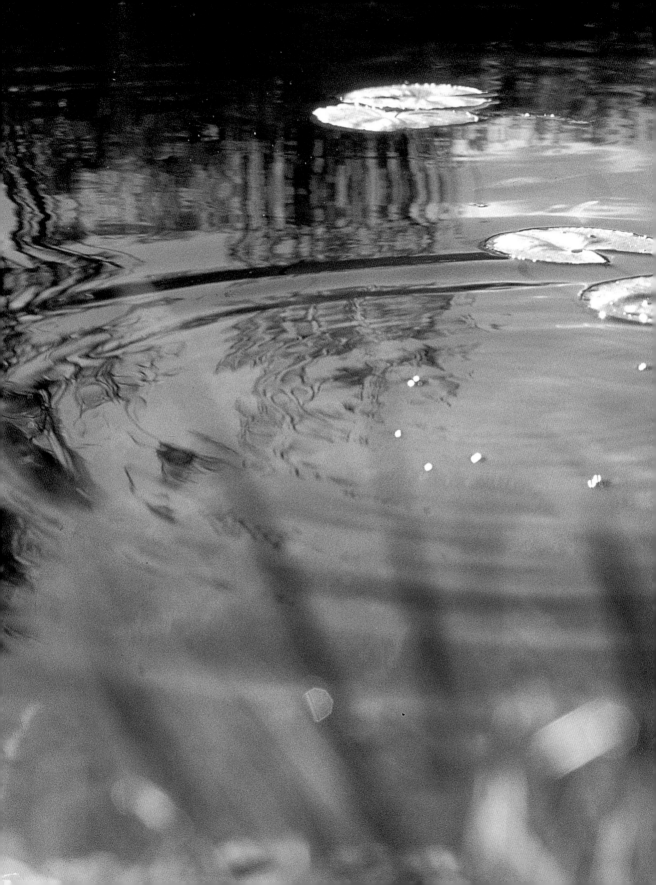

This simple version of a classic and versatile meditation technique helps cleanse your mind by offering a welcome respite from worry. Start by finding a quiet place free from distractions, and sit in a meditative pose on the floor (see page 178 ▶) or in a chair with your feet on the ground, hands resting in your lap or on the arms of the chair. Keep your spine straight, relax your shoulders, and be careful not to let your chin sink down toward your chest. Now close your eyes and take a few deep breaths, inflating your lungs fully as you inhale and emptying them completely as you exhale.

creative visualization

After your breathing has settled into a slow, easy rhythm, begin to visualize a small pond with clear water in a picturesque setting. A bright blue sky stretches overhead, dotted with a few small, fluffy clouds that are reflected on the pond's smooth surface. Picture a pebble falling into the pond. Watch as it slowly sinks through the clear water, down, down, to the bottom. Now imagine that you are that pebble, resting lightly on the bottom of the pond, and look up toward the sky. Imagine that the clouds are your thoughts—all your worries and to-do lists. For a few minutes, just watch them drift past. You know you'll deal with them later, but, for now, your mind is still and unconcerned as you rest contentedly in your watery haven.

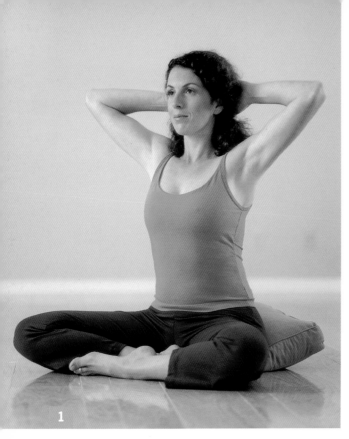

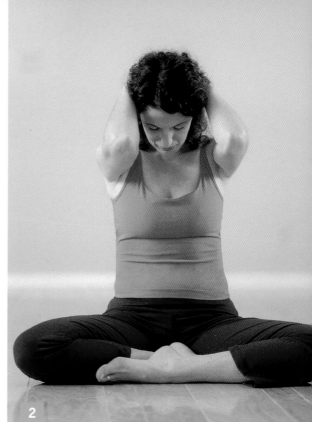

1

2

3

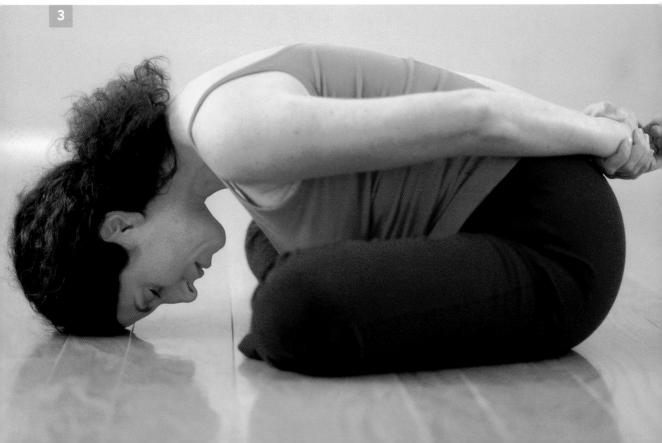

folding wings, yogic seal

Nurture yourself with two cleansing yoga poses that release energy trapped inside your neck, shoulder, and back muscles, helping you find your calm center.

1 To perform Folding Wings, sit cross-legged on the floor, elongate your spine, interlace your fingers, and bring your hands to the back of your head. Inhaling, press your elbows back, careful to exert only gentle pressure on your head, and open your shoulder blades wide.

2 Exhaling, fold your arms alongside your ears, lengthen the back of your neck, and bring your chin toward your chest. Inhale as you lift your head and press your elbows back again. Repeat these opening and closing movements for four breaths.

3 Add to this feeling of release by doing Yogic Seal. Staying in a cross-legged sitting position, bring your hands behind your back and gently grasp the wrist of your dominant hand with your other hand. Inhale and elongate your spine, then exhale as you fold forward from your hips. Keep your hands relaxed against your back. Let your head hang toward or rest against the floor. If this is uncomfortable, place a firm cushion under your head. Direct your mind to a place of utter stillness. Hold for 30 to 60 seconds, then slowly sit up while inhaling.

Just Breathe
Try to pay careful attention to your breathing as you practice these—as well as all other—yoga moves. In yoga, inhalation usually is linked to movements that expand the chest and abdomen, and exhalation is keyed to movements that compress the abdomen. As you hold poses, try to breathe through your nose, and never hold your breath, which can strain your body, unless specifically instructed to do so.

WHAT CAUSES A PAIN IN THE NECK?

The human neck, the longest neck of any primate, supports the weight of the head—nine pounds or more in an adult. It's one of the busiest parts of the human body but is less protected than the rest of the spine. The neck usually does its job admirably when we use proper posture and let our heads rest directly on top of our spines. But too often we engage in bad habits, such as leaning toward a computer screen for hours, making the neck muscles work much harder and exerting enormous pressure on the cervical vertebrae.

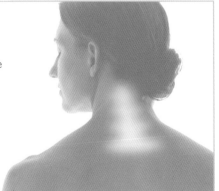

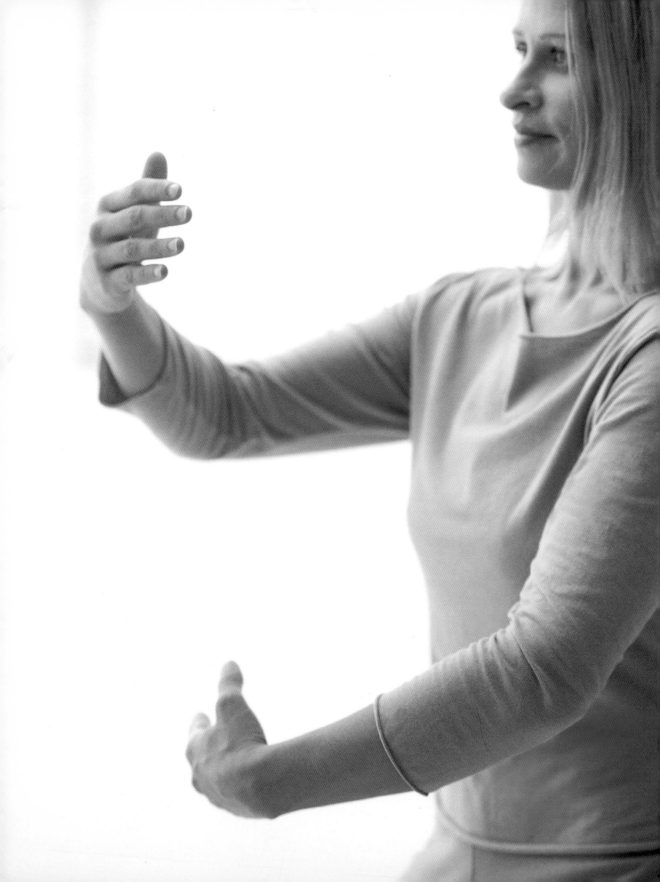

single whip, cloud hands

The circular movements and gentle turns in this tai chi exercise are said to help cleanse and settle the body's organs, especially those of the digestive system.

Tai chi practitioners believe this ancient art cleanses the body and mind in numerous vital ways. The sequence of slow, connected movements keeps the body's *chi* (or life energy) flowing and balanced, which, in turn, can help prevent disease, promote healing, and keep you in harmony with other people and nature. The concentration required to stay aware of the body's movement and energy also helps clear the mind of mental clutter and unwelcome distractions, which fosters clarity and a sense of peacefulness.

The steps outlined on the following pages show you how to move from the Single Whip position into the Cloud Hands sequence. Cloud Hands is also sometimes called Wave Hands Like Clouds or Cloudy Hands. This sequence is a fundamental tai chi form; its graceful circular movements and turns are thought to help connect the upper and lower body, release pent-up tension, and benefit the digestive organs, particularly the stomach.

THE CLEANSING EFFECTS OF TAI CHI

Many practitioners assert that specific tai chi postures directly benefit specific organs, because the positions both physically move the organs and activate energy meridians that correspond to those organs. The movements of Single Whip, Cloud Hands, for instance, are believed to massage the digestive organs, helping to rid them of impurities and make them function more efficiently. In addition, the meditative aspects of tai chi help cleanse the mind of worry and tension, which can reduce the amount of acid secreted into the stomach. In fact, doctors in Asian hospitals often use tai chi as part of their treatment regimen for ulcer patients.

step-by-step sequence ▶

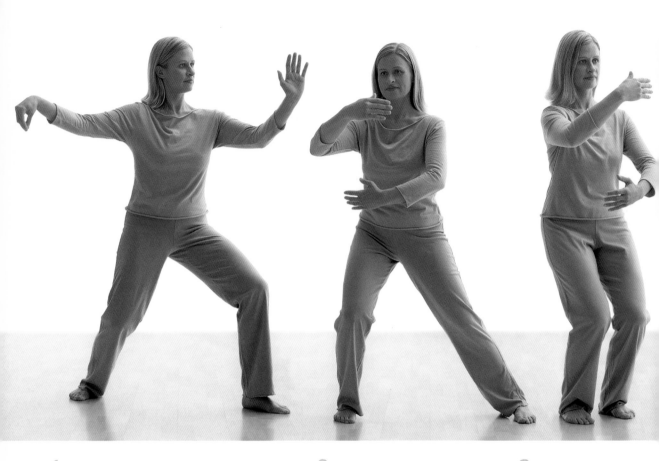

1 Start in the Single Whip position: legs apart, with the left leg in front and bent at the knee and the right leg behind you and almost straight. Your left toes point toward the left, your right toes point slightly toward the right. Raise your arms to a little below shoulder height, with your left arm bent up at the elbow and your palm facing out. Extend your right arm in back of you, with a slight bend at your elbow, and close your fingers gently and point them down (as if you're making a beak or a hook). Relax your shoulders.

2 To move into the Cloud Hands sequence, pivot on your left foot, so that your toes are facing forward and the left leg is extended. Keep your weight on your bent right leg. As you move, draw the left arm down and in, until your hand is near your navel, palm facing in. Draw your right arm up and in so your hand is about chin level and your palm is facing toward you. Keep both arms rounded.

3 Take a step in with your left foot, while keeping your knees bent at about 45 degrees. Remember to keep your knees softly bent throughout the exercise. (When practicing tai chi, always keep the angles of your joints soft, or relaxed.)

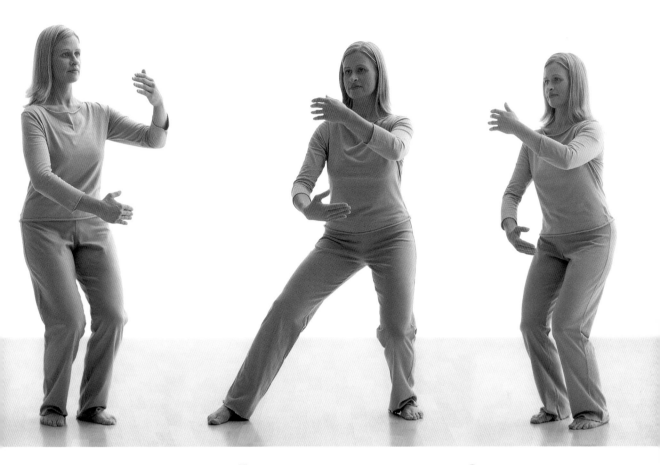

4 Begin to turn at the waist toward the right. In a controlled, flowing motion, exchange hand positions: Your right hand goes down, and your left comes up. Your palms remain facing in and your arms remain rounded, as if you were still holding the barrel.

5 As part of the continuous flow of movement toward the right, extend your right leg out to the side, while keeping the knee softly bent. At the same time, concentrate on putting all of your weight into your left leg. In tai chi parlance, your right leg should feel empty now, while your left (weight-bearing) leg should feel full. Make sure your shoulders continue to stay dropped and relaxed.

6 Take a step in with your right foot, keeping your knees bent softly. Your left hand stays up and your right hand stays down. You can now move back into the Single Whip position (see Step 1) and repeat the sequence four more times.

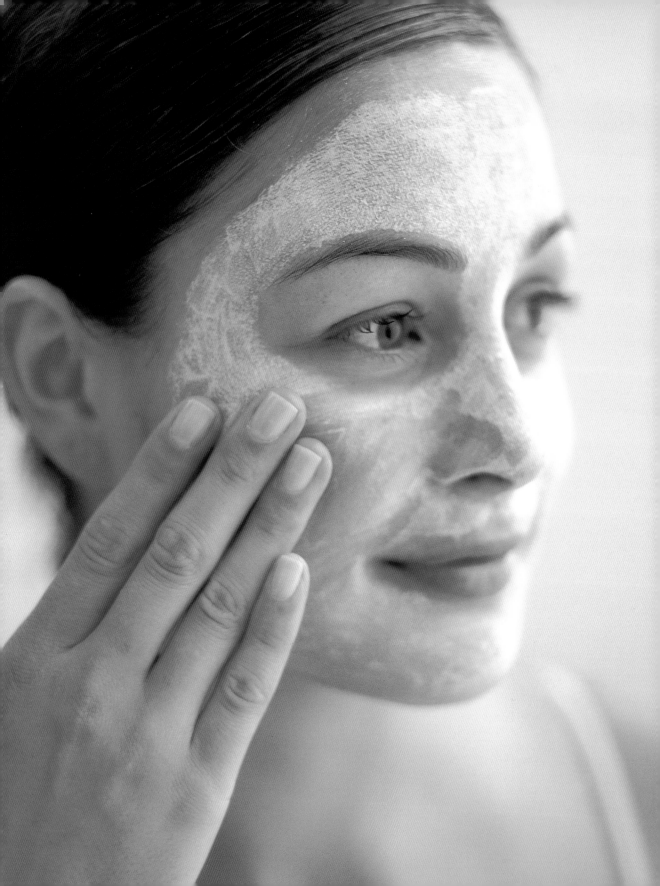

tea tree oil mask

If you have oily or blemish-prone skin, regular use of a deep-cleaning mask made of tea tree oil keeps excess oil under control and breakouts to a minimum.

Oily skin is caused by overzealous sebaceous (oil) glands—or simply an overabundance of them. The greasy film that results can give your skin an unwelcome shine and clog pores, encouraging blemishes and blackheads. Tea tree oil's deep-cleaning properties help combat these problems, and its antibacterial qualities both soothe blemishes and prevent new ones from forming. (Tea tree oil also can help prevent infections in cuts and may alleviate cold sores and sunburns.)

After washing your face, apply a tea tree oil–based facial mask (many excellent commercial products are available, but see the recipe at right for a homemade version). Spread a thin, even layer over your face, avoiding the lip and eye areas. Leave it on for ten minutes. Remove the mask by rinsing your face with warm water and wiping away any residue with a moistened cotton pad or washcloth.

Keep in mind that even oily skin can need moisturizing. A tea tree oil–based moisturizing gel softens and hydrates your skin without being too heavy or irritating. Apply about a quarter-sized squeeze of gel onto clean fingers and massage it into your skin.

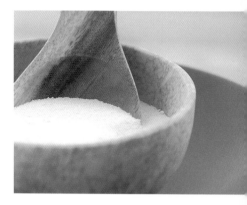

Deep-Cleaning Mask

1½ tablespoons kaolin (white
   clay, pictured above)

1 tablespoon oat flour

3 to 4 tablespoons orange juice

1 tablespoon finely chopped
   mint leaves

1 teaspoon extra-virgin olive oil

5 to 8 drops tea tree oil

KEEPING BLEMISHES AT BAY

Excess oil production, especially in the face's T-zone (forehead, nose, and chin), is the main cause of pimples. While that's a matter of genetics, diet and stress also are believed to play a role. A host of products claim to battle blemishes, but many contain ingredients that are extremely drying to the skin, causing irritation and encouraging the production of even more oil. If you're plagued by pimples, consult a dermatologist to see what treatments the doctor recommends.

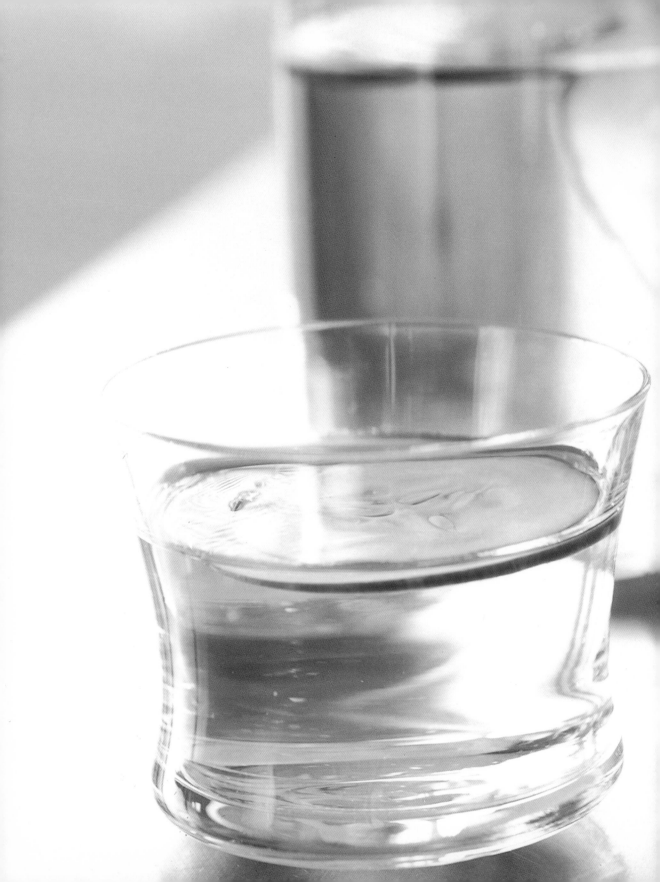

You can find lots of exotic potions on the market touting all sorts of health benefits. But one of the simplest (and least expensive!) ways to cleanse your system is to drink plenty of water. After oxygen, your body needs water more than any other substance; in fact, about half of an adult woman's body is made up of water.

the virtues of water

Water plays an immensely important role in your body's functioning. It makes your skin elastic and supple, and keeps primary systems— such as metabolism, digestion, circulation, and the internal thermostat—working properly. It also lubricates joints and muscles, fights fatigue, and helps flush toxins from your body, preventing undue stress on your kidneys and liver. Even minor dehydration has been linked to faulty concentration and irritability; severe dehydration can be life threatening.

So how much of this magic elixir do you really need? Although scientists don't have a definitive answer yet, the current standard advice is to drink eight glasses of water a day (about 64 ounces)— more if you exercise often or live in a hot climate. If that sounds like an awful lot to consume, remember that it's really 64 ounces of fluid—and fluid includes juice, milk, and herbal teas, as well as the water content in the foods you eat.

forehead sweeps

After cleansing your face, take a moment to give yourself a forehead massage. It aids lymphatic drainage and shifts facial muscles from habitual positions.

Not only does facial massage relieve tension, it actually can enhance your appearance. Massaging improves blood circulation, which helps impart a radiant glow, and it also relaxes the tensed muscles that can give a weary, pinched look to your face.

1 Relax in any comfortable position. Close your eyes, and place the middle finger of each hand on the innermost corners of your eyebrows (the part nearest your nose).

2 Applying gentle but firm pressure, slowly trace a path from just above your eyebrows to your temples. (Firm pressure helps ease muscle tension.) Return to the starting position.

3 Sweep out again, this time moving just below your eyebrows to your temples. Take care to press on the brow bone, not your eyes.

4 For the third pass, trace a path from the innermost corners of your eyebrows up to your hairline. Glide your fingers across your forehead and down to your temples. Complete three sets of sweeps.

Bonus Massage Strokes
To supplement the relaxing effect of the forehead sweeps, release built-up energy around the head by doing a few broad strokes as well. Close your eyes and cover your forehead with one hand, positioning your hand horizontally across your forehead. Lightly stroke up from your eyebrows to the top of your head. Switch hands and repeat. Alternating hands, perform about two dozen strokes.

WHAT CAUSES WRINKLES?

The movement of facial muscles creases the skin, and aging—with its attendant loss of collagen, facial fat, and oil production—can turn those creases into furrows. Add the sun's effects (see page 54 ◄) and smoking (which researchers have found turns on a gene that destroys collagen), and you get your own personal recipe for wrinkles. To help slow down their formation, use sunscreen and moisturizers with antioxidants, don't smoke, and wear sunglasses and hats. Massage also helps ease tense facial muscles, which helps reduce creasing.

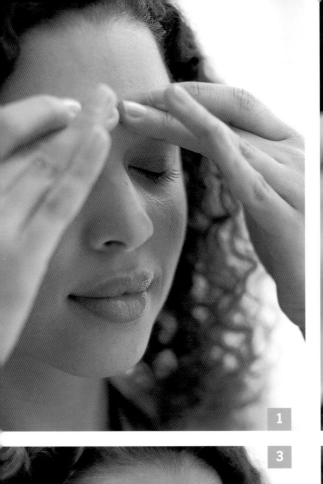

1

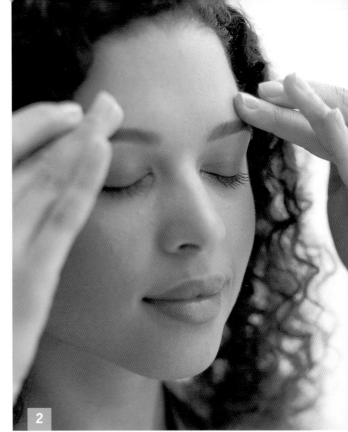

2

3

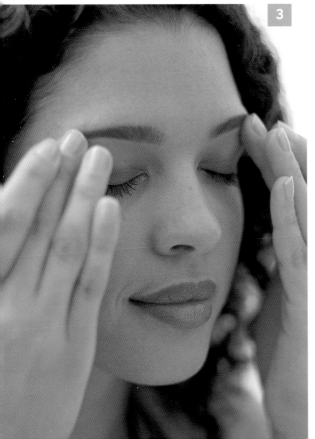

4

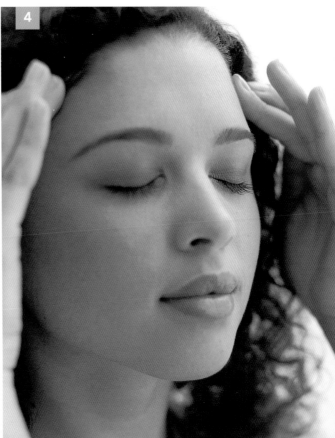

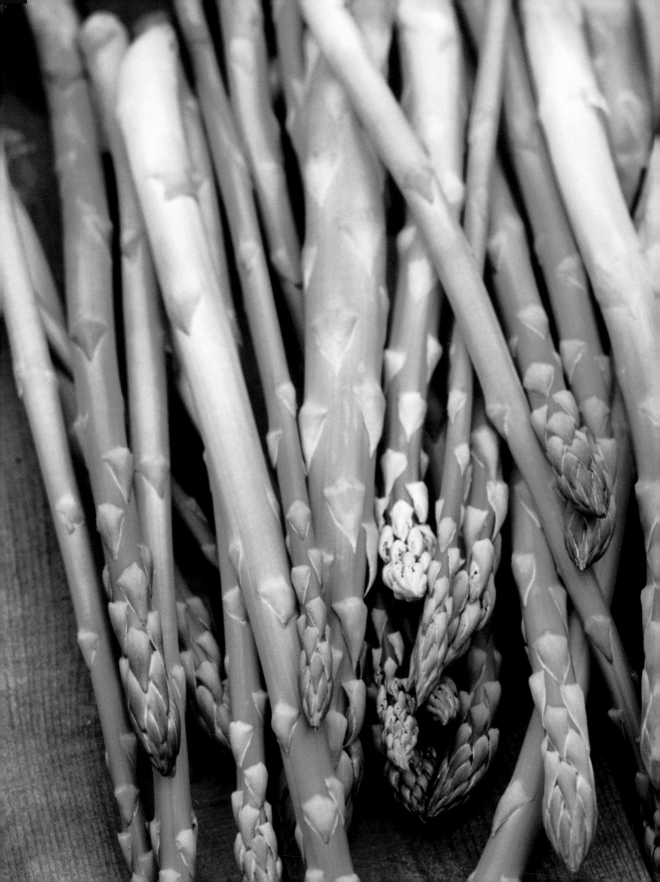

roasted asparagus

A hallmark of spring, tender spears of asparagus lend an elegant touch to any meal. Their healthful properties treat your body to a little spring cleaning, as well.

Asparagus has earned pride of place among vegetables in many cultures for both its taste and its medicinal qualities. In the kitchen, you'll find it giving a flavorful crunch to Italian risotto, simmered with onions and dill to create Russian soups, and paired with black bean sauce in Chinese kitchens. In traditional medicine, asparagus (usually the root) has been used to cure toothaches, prevent kidney stones, retard hair loss, and ward off cancer. A potent diuretic, it helps cleanse the body of excess fluids and naturally occurring toxins.

Fresh asparagus lends itself to many types of preparations, from the sublimely simple (such as steamed and sprinkled with salt and pepper, maybe dressed with a little olive oil) to the elaborate (baked in thin slices of ham and served with a creamy lemon sauce, for example). The recipe here is a good compromise: With the tang provided by the balsamic vinegar and lemon zest, it's easy enough to make for a family meal and sophisticated enough for a formal dinner.

1 Preheat the oven to 400°. Line a low-sided roasting pan with aluminum foil and pour the olive oil in the middle of the pan.

2 Pat the asparagus spears dry and roll them in the olive oil to coat them. Season to taste with salt and pepper.

3 Roast the asparagus for 20 to 25 minutes, turning the spears two or three times during roasting. The asparagus is done when the spears can be pierced with a fork (be careful not to overcook them).

4 Place the asparagus spears on a serving dish. Drizzle with the balsamic vinegar, turning the spears to coat them well. Garnish with the lemon zest. Serve warm or at room temperature.

Ingredients

2 teaspoons extra-virgin olive oil

1 pound large fresh asparagus spears, trimmed and cut into 1-inch pieces

Kosher salt and freshly ground pepper

2 teaspoons balsamic vinegar

Finely grated lemon zest for garnish

- Serves: 4
- Prep time: 10 minutes
- Cook time: 20 to 25 minutes

Nutritional Information Per Serving
Aspartic acid and potassium give asparagus its diuretic qualities.

Calories	40
Kilojoules	170
Protein	3 g
Carbohydrates	3 g
Total Fat	2.5 g
Saturated Fat	0.5 g
Cholesterol	0 mg
Sodium	2 mg
Dietary Fiber	1 g

strengthen

Not so long ago, many women wanted to appear
dainty and delicate. But today, women are much
more likely to celebrate the virtues of a strong body,
a keen and focused mind, and a resilient spirit.

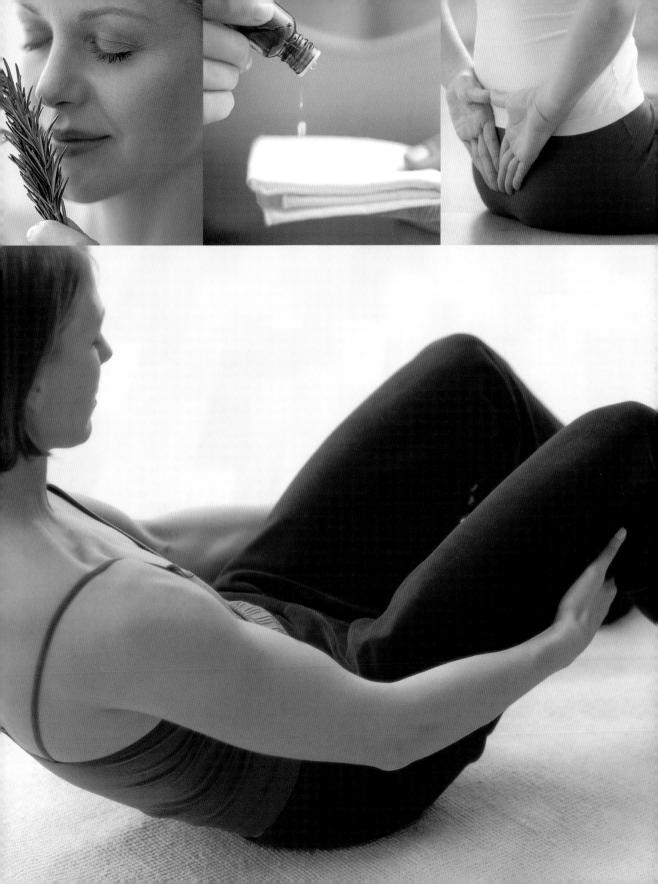

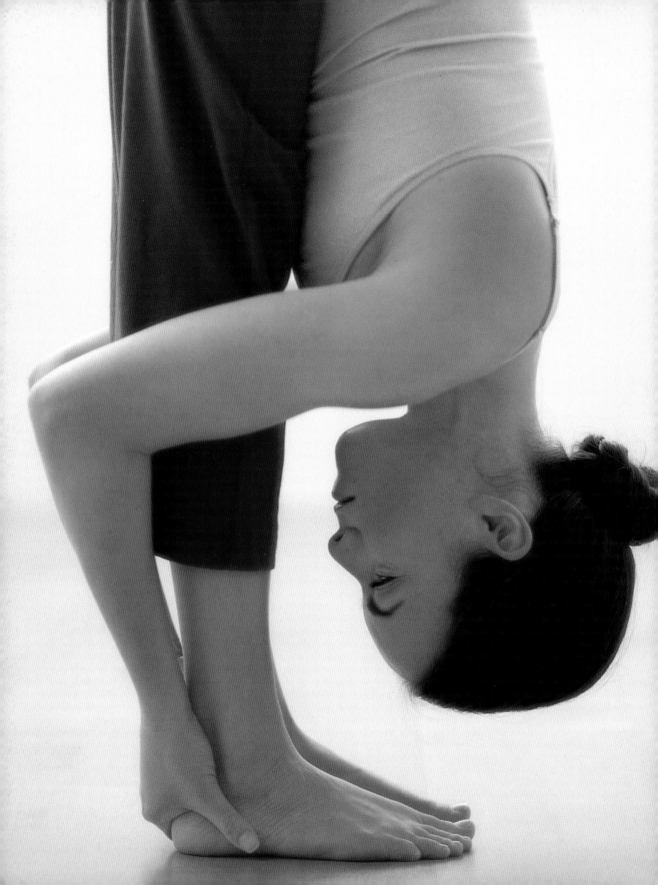

strengthen

When someone is described as a strong woman, what image comes to mind? An accomplished athlete, a hard-driving executive, a pillar of the family? All, of course, are valid interpretations of the phrase, and they certainly aren't mutually exclusive, as women wear many hats these days and need to be strong in a variety of ways.

Being strong not only lets you get more out of life now, it helps ward off some of the common pitfalls of aging. It's a sad fact that, as early as our mid-20s, we start losing some of our muscle tone—by age 74 or so, 66 percent of all women can't even lift a gallon of milk. But it doesn't have to be that way. Working out with weights and doing weight-bearing exercises such as running and aerobics holds that muscle loss at bay. Those strong muscles, in turn, help reduce the amount of body fat you would otherwise accumulate as you age, and prevent injuries to knees, hips, and backs. Weight-bearing exercises also help you avoid the ravages of osteoporosis in later life. And since, no matter what your age, staying strong means having an alert mind and a buoyant spirit, you'll also find ideas on these pages to help empower you in these vital realms as well.

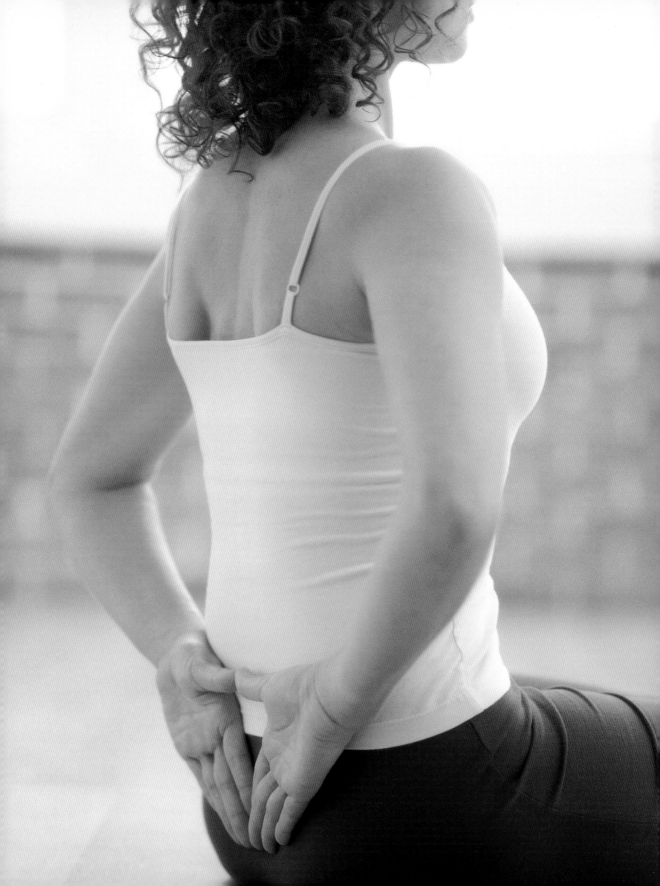

tummy tighteners

This series of abdominal-strengthening yoga poses lets you gradually increase the intensity of your workout as you gain muscle tone and confidence.

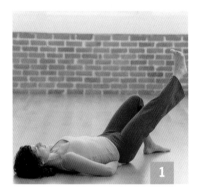
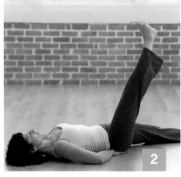
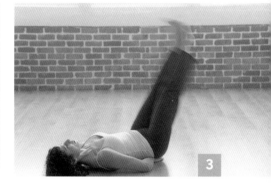

Throughout these poses, use the Diamond Base position (pictured at left) to keep your back supported. Place your hands against your lower back, palms out, with the tips of your thumbs and index fingers touching. Remember to also press your lower back down firmly. If your back lifts up—a sign that you're straining it—stop and rest.

1 Lie on your back and place your left foot on the floor so your bent left knee points upward. Keeping your right leg straight and your foot flexed, inhale as you lift your leg as high as is comfortable (no more than 90 degrees). As you exhale, lower your leg, keeping your foot flexed. Do this six times, then repeat with your other leg.

2 To make this basic lift a little more challenging, keep your resting leg straight along the floor as you work the other leg. Alternate legs, lifting each leg six times. Remember to build intensity gradually; if you feel any strain, go back to the easier version.

3 When you're ready, you can increase your workout by holding your resting leg straight up toward the ceiling while you lift and lower the other leg. Work each leg six times.

Tight Abs for Life

Vanity might motivate you to work those abs, but strong abdominals are actually vital to your overall health and fitness. They take some strain off your back, aid digestion, and can help relieve menstrual pain. They might even help you live longer: A recent Canadian study compared the strength, flexibility, and exercise habits of 8,116 people and tracked their mortality rate over 13 years. The one factor that correlated with a higher death rate? Having weak abdominal muscles.

brush knee

In this tai chi movement, the subtle force of shifting your weight helps you develop balance, agility, and strength. Work slowly to gain the maximum benefit.

Building Muscles, Tai Chi Style

The slow, flowing movements of tai chi might look as if they provide little challenge to muscles. But because you do the exercises in a crouching position and shift your balance from one leg to another, you build strong leg muscles, while avoiding the risks of high-impact exercise. The twisting and turning in tai chi also help develop your abdominal muscles.

1 Begin with your legs together and slightly bent. Your right foot should be in back of your left and the heel should be up; keep your left foot firmly planted on the floor. Raise your hands to chin level, with your fingers parted and facing outward. Your left hand should be close to your head; your right arm should be extended, with the elbow bent slightly. Look out over your right hand.

2 Step out with your right foot, keeping both feet flat. Tai chi instructors say that your left leg should feel "full" (that is, it should be bearing most of your weight); your right leg should feel "empty."

3 Lower your right arm, bending your elbow slightly and keeping your palm flat and facing the ground. Push out with your left hand, with your fingers pointing up. As always in tai chi, try to keep your joints—wrists, knees, elbows, and so on—relaxed, with soft angles, as you move. When you're done, you can repeat these steps on the other side, and then alternate both sides again.

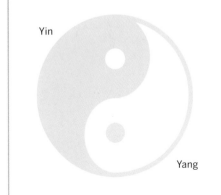

Yin

Yang

A BALANCE OF FORCES

The yin–yang symbol illustrated at left depicts the principle that lies at the very heart of the ancient practice of tai chi: the constant interplay between what seem to be opposing universal energies. The dark half of the circle represents *yin* (a passive, receptive, feminine, and still energy); the light half represents *yang* (an active, creative, masculine, and moving energy). Translated into physical movements, inhalation and yielding embody the yin, while exhalation and thrusting embody the yang. Yin and yang are complementary. Indeed, the "seeds"—or dots within the two halves—emphasize that the potential for yang is implicit in yin, and vice versa.

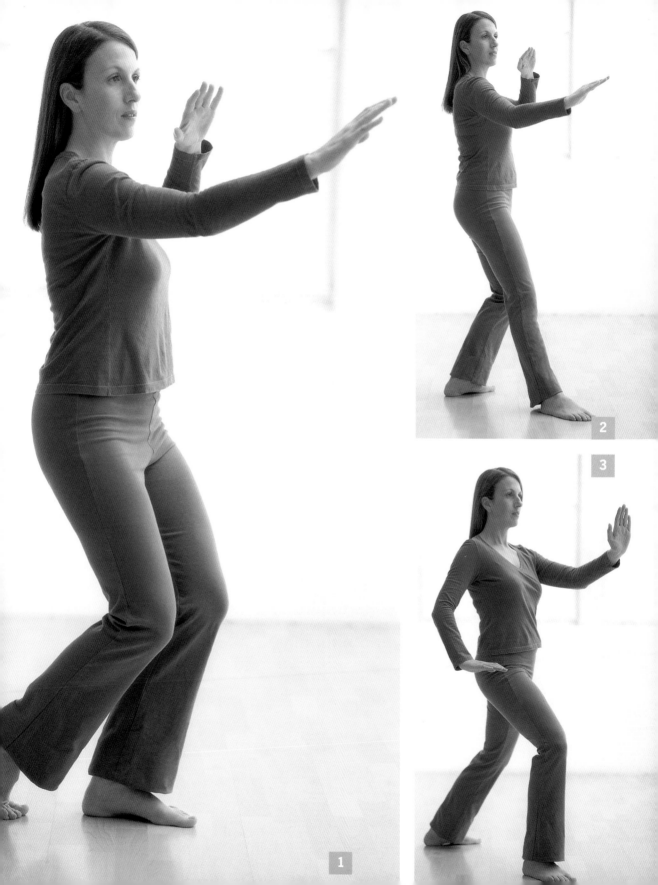

1

2

3

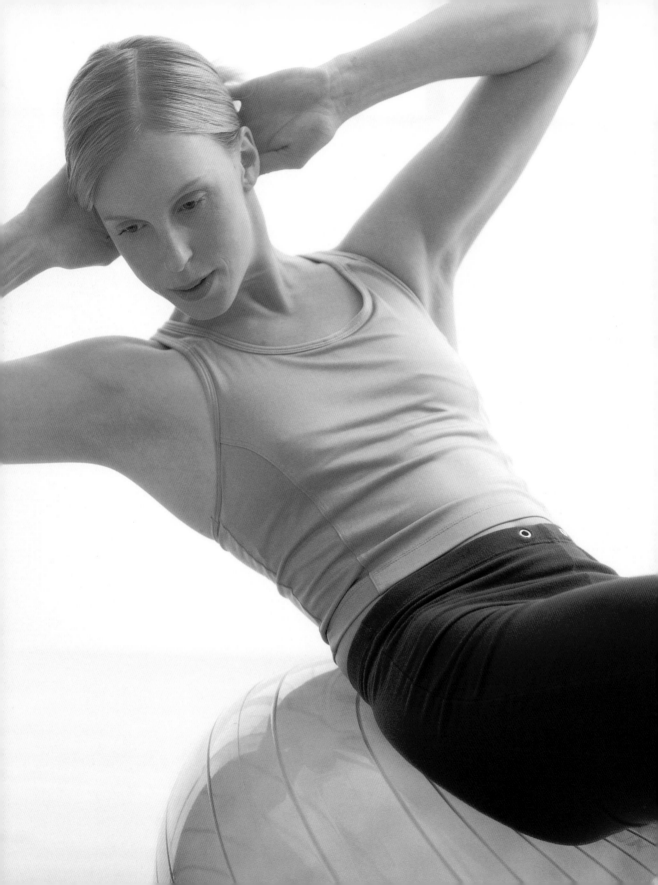

rosemary workout

Enhance your morning run, your session at the gym, or your game of tennis by incorporating invigorating aromatherapy into your exercise routine.

The next time you head out to exercise, tuck a new accessory into your gym bag: a handkerchief sprinkled with rosemary essential oil. Aromatherapists claim that inhaling rosemary's invigorating scent before working out helps enhance concentration and combat fatigue. The camphoraceous aroma lets you breathe more easily and deeply, thus increasing oxygen flow in your body.

Using this form of aromatherapy-on-the-go couldn't be simpler: Just put a drop or two of rosemary essential oil on a clean handkerchief, place it in a sealable plastic bag, and take it out just prior to working out. Keeping your eyes closed (so the vapors don't irritate them), open the bag and breathe in deeply for 20 seconds or so. You'll feel the rousing effect of the rosemary almost immediately.

Rosemary has many other uses in the locker room, too. A massage-oil blend containing rosemary essential oil can stimulate circulation, for example. And after a workout, a rosemary rubdown or bath can soothe tense, aching muscles—and lift your spirits.

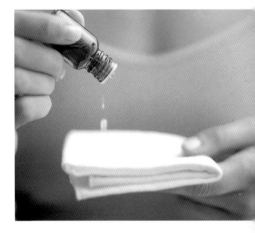

Other Stimulating Options

When it comes to the right essential oil to carry in your gym bag, rosemary is often touted as the ultimate pick-me-up scent. But if rosemary isn't your scent of choice, aromatherapists also recommend other essential oils to enhance physical and mental performance, including eucalyptus, peppermint, and Spanish marjoram.

PUTTING THE BRAIN ON ALERT

Can the scent of an essential oil affect the brain? Science says yes. A U.S. research team found that people who smelled rosemary oil for three minutes showed increased alertness, less anxiety, and an ability to do math problems faster (though not more accurately) than before their aromatherapy treatment. And British researchers found that people who sniffed lavender oil or no oil were less alert and had more difficulty with memory tasks than those who smelled rosemary essential oil before taking the researchers' tests.

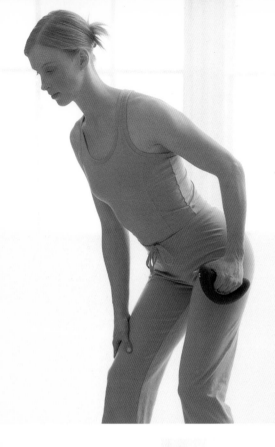

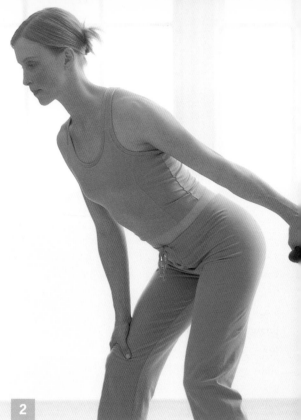

1

2

3

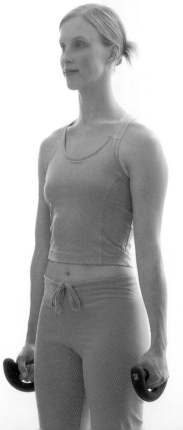

4

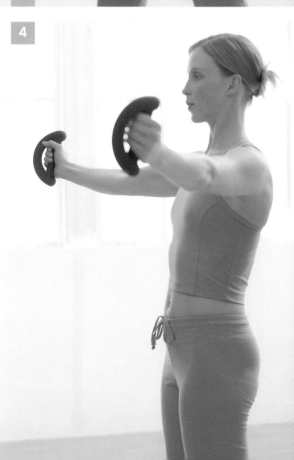

basic arm exercises

Arm muscles are among the most obliging in the body, responding quickly to exercise. Just perform these moves every other day for a few weeks and you'll see.

1 Stand tall, holding a weight in your left hand. Then step out with your right leg and bend your knee; position your knee in line with your second toe. Rest your right hand on your thigh, just above your bent right knee. Your left leg remains comfortably in back of you, with your toes facing straight ahead and your knee slightly bent. Draw in your abdominal muscles, as if you were pulling your navel toward your spine. Make sure your shoulders and hips are square, angle your tailbone slightly up, and keep your neck straight as you gaze directly at the floor. Lift your left upper arm in line with your torso, ensuring your elbow is bent about 90 degrees.

2 With your upper body and legs as still as possible, on the exhale, straighten your arm, pivoting from the elbow. Keep your wrist straight and upper arm stable and along the same line as your torso. Bend your arm to return to the starting position. Repeat 15 times. To help you establish the correct rhythm, raise your arm up for two counts, hold for one, and slowly lower down for four counts. Then, holding the weight in your right hand and bending your left leg forward, repeat this exercise 15 times with your right hand.

3 Now, holding a weight in each hand, stand up straight with your feet hip-width apart and your arms resting at your sides. Your toes should be pointed straight ahead, your shoulders down and back, and your knees slightly bent. Draw in your abs and look straight ahead.

4 On the exhale, raise both of your arms, thumbs up, at a 30-degree angle out from your body until your hands reach eye level. Keep your shoulder blades down and collarbones wide, and don't let your back arch. Hold for one count and then, on the inhale, return your arms slowly to the starting position. Repeat this step 10 times. (If your muscles get sore after exercising, try the massage on page 126 ▸.)

A Weighty Matter

Incorporating free weights into your exercise routine is key to maximizing your results. To make sure that you don't strain your wrists and arm muscles, start with weights that feel good in your hands, ergonomically speaking. They should seem fairly light at first but should challenge you as you perform a number of repetitions. As you gain strength, move on to a heavier set of weights (for example, from three pounds to five and then to eight). The last three repetitions should always feel a bit challenging but not so difficult that you can't maintain good form.

basic leg exercises

This sequence works the glutes, hamstrings, quads, and lower legs, while honing your balance and the weight-shifting skills critical in skiing and other sports.

1 Stand up straight with your legs slightly wider than hip-width apart, hands at your sides. Tuck in your chin slightly, distribute your body weight evenly between the balls of your feet and heels; tighten your abdominals by drawing your belly button toward your spine.

2 On an inhale, squat: Drop your butt back and fold at the break of your legs. Lift your chest and extend your arms in front of you for balance. Bring your thighs as parallel to the floor as is comfortable, but do not strain. Aim your knees over the second toe of each foot.

3 Now come out of the squat, pushing off from your heels as you exhale and lowering your arms as you rise. Just as you are back up to a standing position, lift your right leg off the floor and extend it 10 degrees behind your body while balancing on your left leg. Keep your spine lengthened and your abs tight; squeeze the right glute. Then bring the leg back to the floor and begin another squat; this time lift your left leg back as you rise up. Alternate legs until you have completed ten repetitions on each leg, for a total of 20 squats. (If your legs get sore after exercising, try the massage on page 129 ▸.)

Exercise Alone Won't Do It

Think you can get rid of the fat on your thighs or tummy with spot exercises? Think again. Exercising or lifting weights will strengthen and tone muscles in those areas, but it won't make the fat go away. (If you build muscle under a fatty deposit, it may make the fat bulge out more!) To get rid of subcutaneous layers of fat, you have to lose weight.

DO WOMEN GAIN WEIGHT AS THEY AGE?

Yes, women typically gain weight as they age because their basal metabolic rate (BMR)—the number of calories burned in a day simply by being alive—drops as muscle mass naturally converts to fat. Since muscles burn eight times as many calories as fat, losing muscle mass reduces your BMR. To counter this process, create (or enhance) an aerobic exercise routine so that you'll burn more calories and do strength training to keep your muscle-to-fat ratio up.

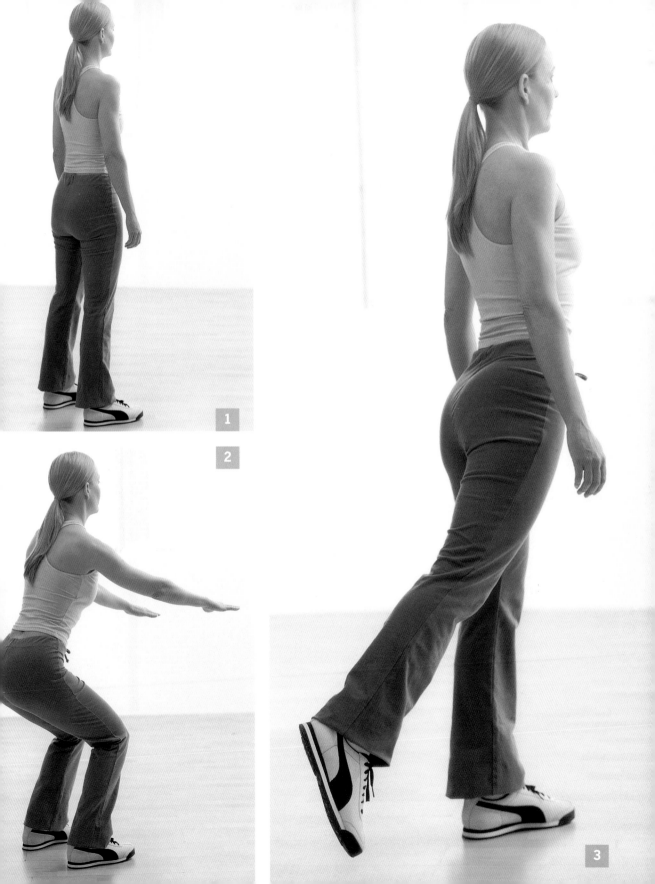

1

2

3

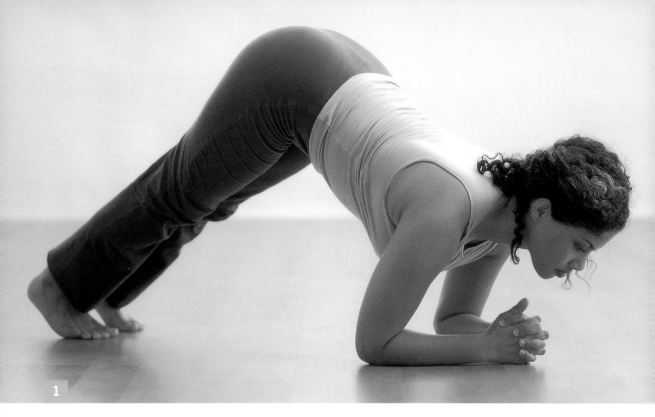

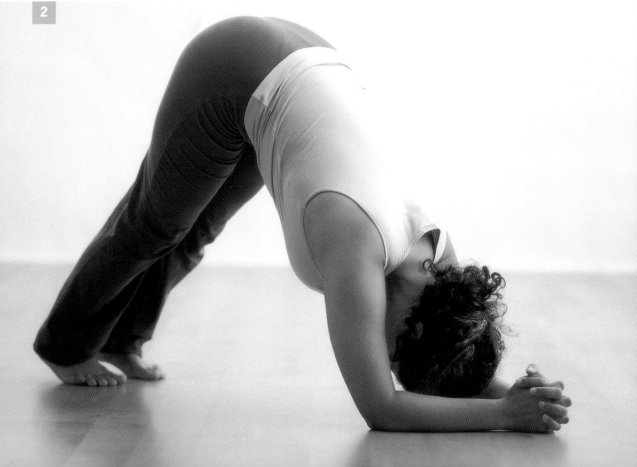

dolphin

This challenging yoga pose, reminiscent of the graceful arc of a dolphin's body, helps strengthen muscles in your arms, upper back, shoulders, and neck.

The Dolphin pose helps build upper-body strength and provides a pleasant stretch for the back muscles that run along your spine. It also promotes neck strength, which is vital for preparing for headstands and other demanding *asanas,* or poses.

1 To get into position, kneel down and grasp each of your upper arms with the opposite hand. Then, still grasping your upper arms, place your elbows on the floor. Keeping your elbows where they are, release your hands and interlace your fingers; lower your forearms to the floor. Make sure that your elbows are slightly closer together than your shoulders are. Next, simultaneously press down with your arms, as if you're trying to push the floor away from your chest, and lift your hips as pictured. Lengthen your spine and allow your head to hang down. Keeping your back straight, inhale and extend your head past your hands, reaching forward with your chin.

2 Exhale and press your chest toward your feet so that your head comes inside your arms. Let your neck relax. Move back and forth between the positions as many times as your comfort level allows.

When Is Enough Enough?
You have to do less stretching than you may think to stay limber and strong. According to many fitness experts, you have to stretch for only ten minutes three or more days a week to start realizing the benefits of these useful exercises.

STRETCH FOR SUCCESS

It's tempting to think that you're fit if you're strong and in good aerobic shape. But the third leg of any fitness program is flexibility. Muscles that are short or stiff are more prone to injury, as are the joints near those muscles. On the other hand, lengthened muscles and joints with a good range of motion (both of which come from stretching) withstand trauma more easily and perform better in both competitive sports and daily activities.

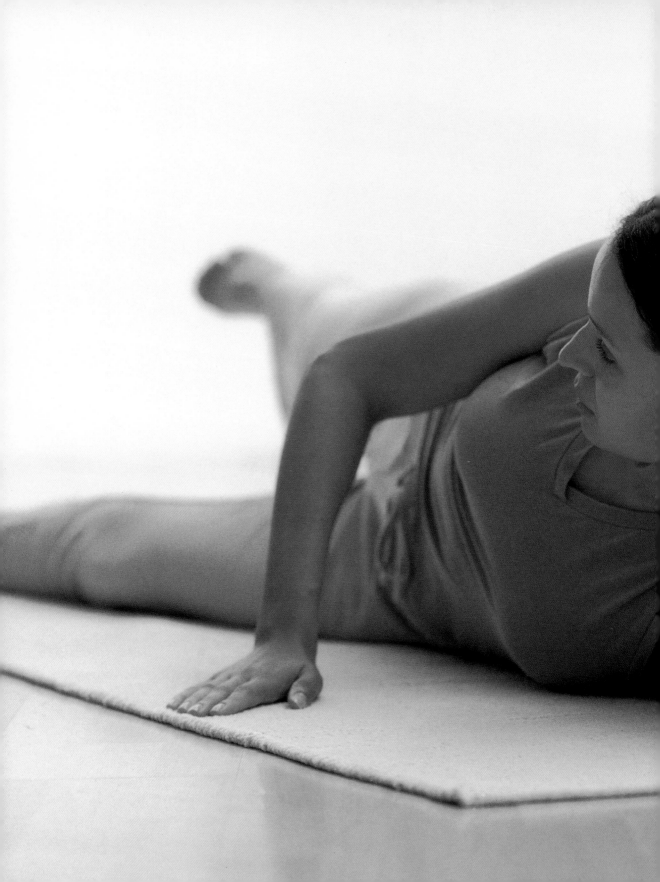

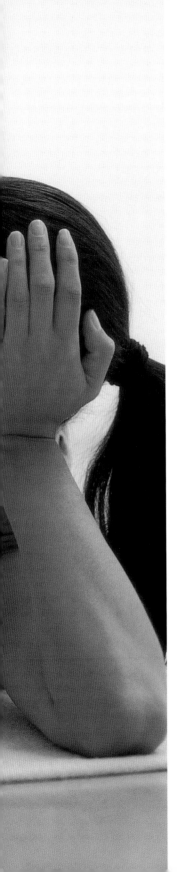

working core muscles

Pilates routines help tone your abdomen, back, and hips by focusing on lengthening and strengthening muscles, rather than using quick, abrupt contractions.

When Joseph Pilates first invented his exercise technique in the 1920s, he didn't call it Pilates. He called it "contrology," because it helped participants develop fine control of their muscles, especially the deep—or core—muscles of the abdomen, back, and buttocks. In fact, Pilates practitioners like to say that the system strengthens muscles from the inside out, rather than the outside in.

The following sequence of Pilates exercises helps develop muscles in the abdomen, back, and hips—areas many women need to strengthen to develop better balance and greater flexibility (not to mention for appearance's sake). The first exercise requires you to synchronize opposite arms and legs, which also helps you improve coordination. Concentrate on the extension—as well as the contraction—in each movement to avoid arching your back, and be sure to keep your navel pulled back toward your spine as you work. Also, keep the abdominals active as you lie on your stomach to help prevent excessive compression of the lower back. (For an even more intense core-muscle workout, try Pilates with a fitness ball; see page 303 ▶.)

WHY THE EMPHASIS ON CORE MUSCLES?

Pilates exercises focus on the muscles that lie deep within the center of the body—muscles known as the "powerhouse" in Pilates circles—including the abdominal, back, buttock, and thigh muscles. Realigning, strengthening, and lengthening these core muscles improves posture, increases circulation, reduces the risk of injury, enables greater range of motion, promotes flexibility, and can even help stave off incontinence. These benefits help account for the skyrocketing popularity of Pilates throughout the world.

step-by-step sequence ▶

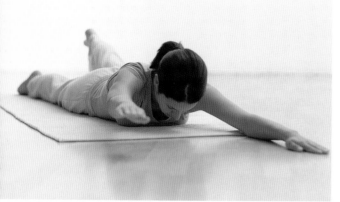

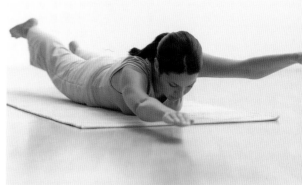

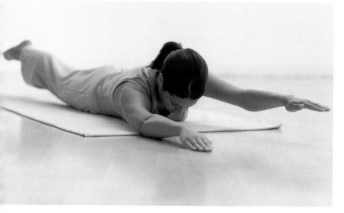

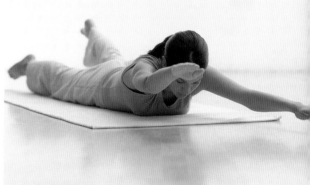

1 This exercise is called "swimming." Lie on your stomach, with your arms straight over your head, feet hip-width apart. Lift your head but look down; keep your neck and spine long, abs pulled in, and feet pointed. Inhale and lift one arm and the opposite leg up about eight inches. Stretch the raised limbs out. Exhale and lower.

2 Inhale and lift the opposite arm and leg, stretch the lifted limbs out, and then lower them. Alternate sides for two to three minutes.

3 To make this a more advanced exercise, lift both of your arms and legs off the ground. Alternate moving opposite arms and legs in a swimming motion.

4 As you get stronger at this exercise, speed up the swimming motion. If your back hurts or you are straining, go back to the simple, alternating swimming movement, with two limbs on the floor at all times.

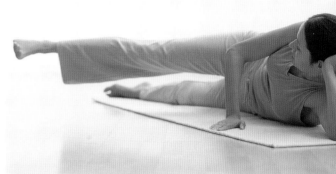

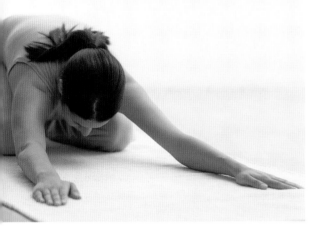

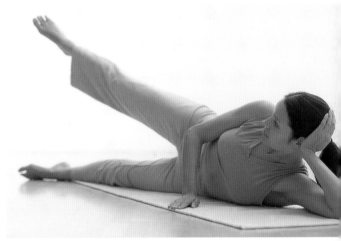

5 Now relax your back by going into what's known as a prayer stretch: Sit back over your heels, with your knees slightly apart, your chest relaxed and close to the floor, and your arms stretched out comfortably in front. Hold this position for about 20 seconds, breathing deeply but naturally the whole time.

6 Lie on your side. Support your head with one arm; place the other in front of you. Lift the top leg a few inches and swing it forward with a flexed foot. Then swing the leg back about ten degrees; point your toes. Keep your torso still. Do eight times with each leg.

7 Lift your top leg up and down, with the leg slightly turned out and toes pointed. Repeat the leg lifts eight times on each side.

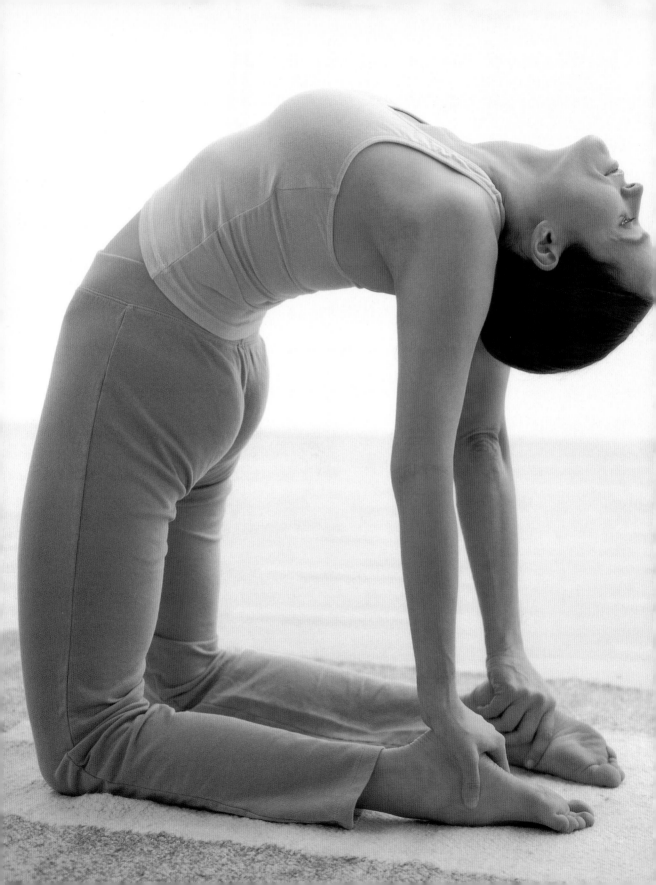

---

victory breath

This classic yoga breathing technique helps you gather steadiness and strength, a useful practice when you're trying to move into more challenging yoga poses.

For more advanced yoga poses, such as the one pictured at left, use the Victory Breath (a breathing technique called *Ujjayi* in Sanskrit) to help you strengthen and stabilize both your mind and body.

First, settle into a comfortable sitting position on the floor or on a rolled-up towel. Exhale slowly through your nose as you gently contract the top of your throat. This involves the same muscular movement in your throat as when you exhale through your mouth to fog up a mirror; you're just doing it with your mouth closed. (In yoga, breathing is almost always done with the mouth closed.) Inhale slowly and deeply, continuing to keep the throat slightly constricted. Listen for a faint hissing sound. (If your breath catches in your throat like a snore, you're contracting the throat too much.)

Use the focus required when practicing the Victory Breath to steady your mind and your body while entering into or holding any pose, particularly those you find challenging.

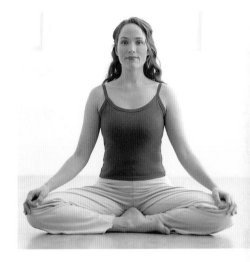

Breathe and Balance
Breathing techniques can help you work through more challenging yoga poses. It's also important to balance *tapas* ("heat" in Sanskrit), the practice of asceticism and discipline for growth, and *ahimsa* ("non-harming"), the principle of caring for yourself and others. Too much tapas manifests itself in physical strain. Strive for a point of maximum effort without strain.

NO PAIN, NO GAIN?

It's common in yoga classes to get a little competitive about the poses—beginners, especially, often want to prove that they're just as flexible or have as much endurance as the veterans in the class, or sometimes even the teachers. How do you tell if you're pushing too hard? Classic signs of strain during your yoga session include trembling, ragged breathing (or a tendency to hold your breath), dizziness, anxiety, and sharp or sudden discomfort. Remember, the idea in yoga is to move slowly, gently, and with awareness—not to be better than your fellow yogis. Measure your ability by your own improvement, not the performance of others.

strengthen

sardines with basil oil

Drizzled with aromatic oil infused with fresh basil, this simple, Mediterranean-inspired dish packs a wallop of bone-strengthening calcium.

Ingredients

2 cups fresh basil leaves,
   stems removed
1½ teaspoons fresh lemon juice
1 cup extra-virgin olive oil, plus
   about 4 tablespoons for brushing
Kosher salt and freshly ground pepper
12 fresh sardines, scaled and gutted

- Serves: 4
- Prep time: 25 minutes
- Cook time: 5 minutes

Nutritional Information Per Serving
Fresh sardines are tastier, but the canned sardines pack more calcium.

Calories	270
Kilojoules	1,140
Protein	12 g
Carbohydrates	1 g
Total Fat	23 g
Saturated Fat	6 g
Cholesterol	70 mg
Sodium	80 mg
Dietary Fiber	0 g

1 Set aside a bowl of ice water. Bring a medium-size pot of salted water to a boil. Add the basil leaves and cook about half a minute, until the leaves are just wilted. Drain, plunge in the ice water, drain again, and squeeze out as much water as possible.

2 Put the basil and lemon juice in a food processor bowl. With the processor running, add the olive oil in a slow, thin stream. When all of the oil has been blended in, season to taste with salt and pepper. Let the mixture stand for 30 minutes at room temperature.

3 Season the sardines lightly with salt. Refrigerate for 30 minutes.

4 Strain the infused oil mixture into a bowl through a sieve lined with dampened cheesecloth. Use a wooden spoon to push all the liquid through the sieve. If the oil is not clear, strain it a second time.

5 Preheat an indoor or outdoor grill to high heat. Brush the sardines with olive oil. Grill the fish for two to three minutes on each side, until just opaque. Drizzle with the basil oil and serve immediately.

BE KIND TO YOUR BONES

Calcium's role in preventing osteoporosis (bone loss) is well known, but researchers now also credit it with helping to ward off heart disease and stroke. Dairy products are the best dietary sources, but other calcium powerhouses include dark leafy vegetables such as kale and mustard greens; almonds and other nuts; calcium-fortified cereals and juices; and seafood such as shrimp, salmon, lobster, and trout. For a snack, try canned sardines; with their soft, edible bones, they offer even more calcium than the fresh variety.

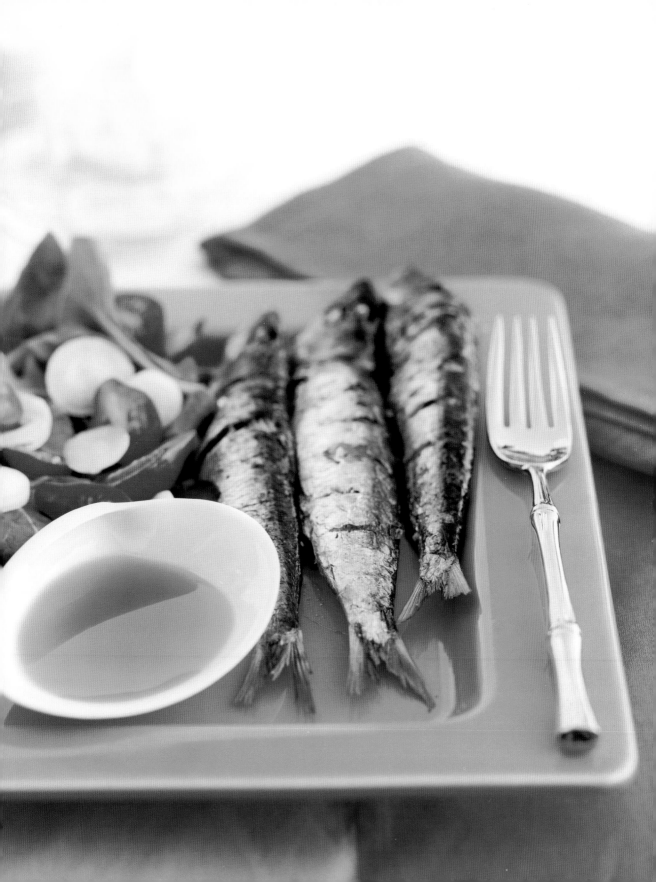

detox

Your mind is sluggish, you feel stressed all the time, you catch one cold after another, and you have the energy of a banana slug. If these symptoms sound familiar, it might be time for a little detoxification.

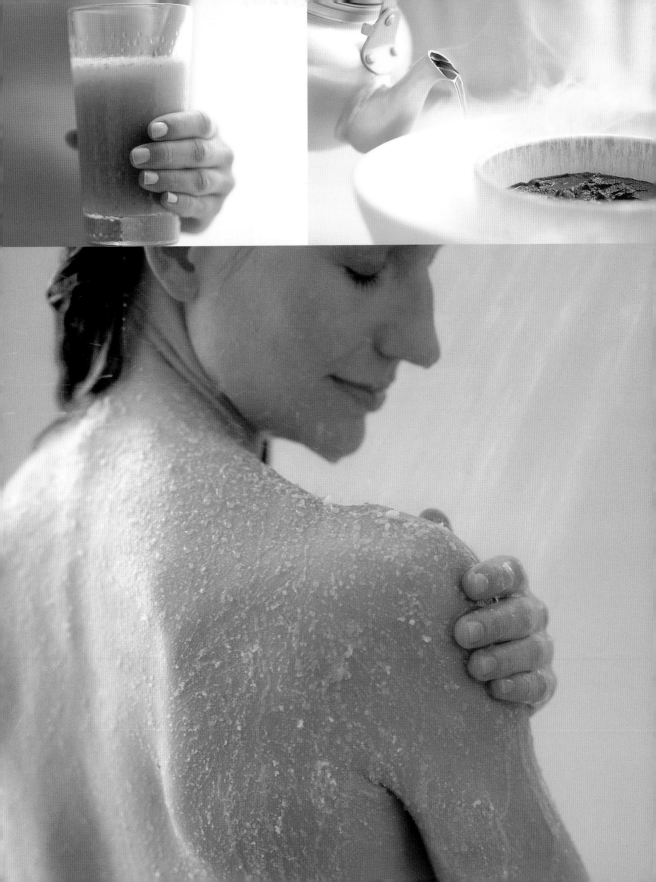

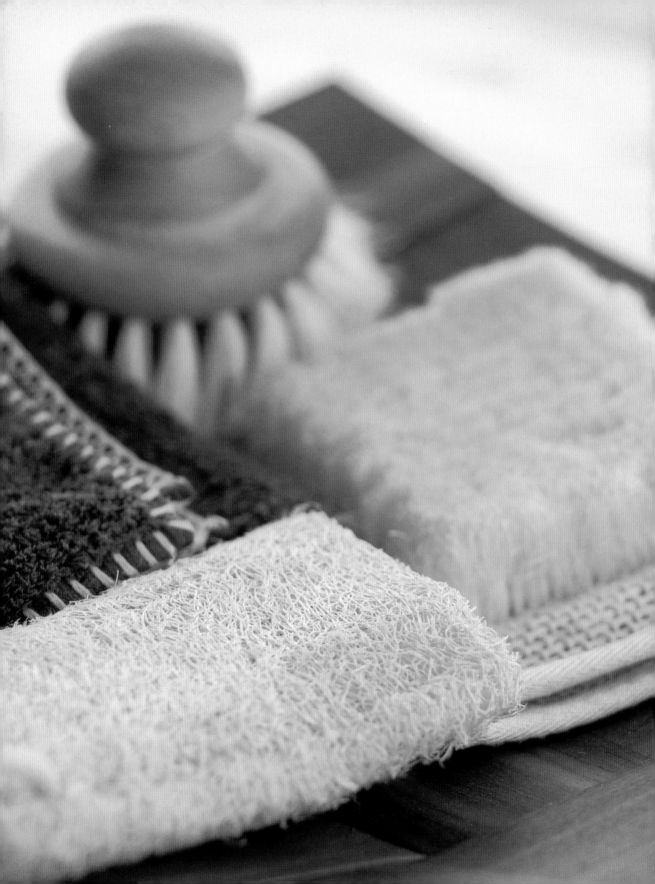

detox

Our bodies do a remarkable job of protecting us from toxins. Our lungs expel carbon dioxide and airborne irritants, and our skin blocks environmental toxins. Lymphatic and circulatory systems, as well as organs such as the liver, kidneys, and bowels, eliminate harmful foreign substances and naturally occurring waste products. But thanks to everything from pollution to our own bad habits, our bodies can't always keep up. When toxins accumulate, they can impair bodily functions, sap our energy, and even make us more susceptible to illnesses and allergies. Sometimes we can see their effects—a dull complexion, dry hair, or a lack of sparkle in the eyes.

That's where detoxification comes in. Detoxing has become trendy, as athletes, film stars, and fitness junkies tout the joys of purging and purifying. But don't let skepticism about the latest colonic fad or extreme detox diet deter you from seeing the real need to help rid your body—and mind—of some of the harmful substances it may be harboring. This chapter isn't meant to be viewed as a total detoxification plan—that usually involves a drastic, if temporary, modification of diet and lifestyle—but you'll find small, helpful steps that are sure to make a difference in how you look and feel.

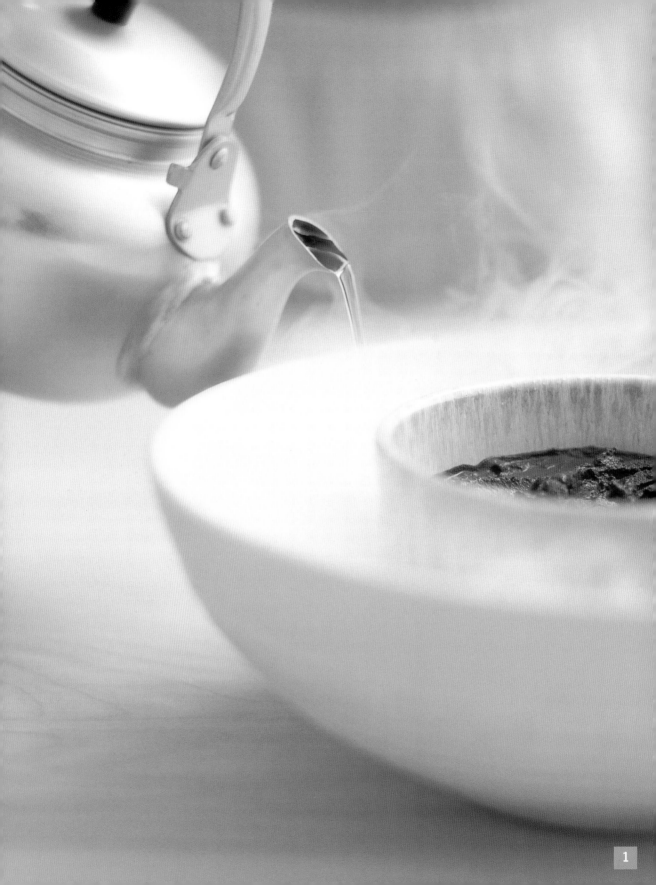

mud pack

When a full-body mud bath isn't a practical option, using a spot pack is a convenient, effective way to reap some of mud's natural healing and detoxifying benefits.

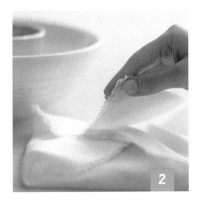
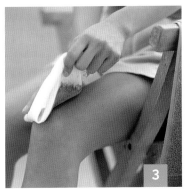

Soothing Mud Pack

1 cup thick, therapeutic body mud
1 small heat-conductive bowl
1 large bowl
Boiling water
1 12-by-12-inch square of
   highly porous cloth
Spatula
Plastic wrap
Towel

How Does Mud Help?

The mud pack's warmth eases aches and pains, while the minerals, vitamins, and plant substances found in therapeutic muds are believed to be absorbed through the skin, clearing metabolic pathways and improving waste elimination, cell oxygenation, and nerve function.

1 To make a mud pack, use a thick, therapeutic body mud (it should not be runny). Scoop about one cup of the mud into a small heat-conductive bowl. Fill a larger bowl two-thirds full with boiling water. Place the bowl of mud into the bowl of water, being careful not to let the water overflow into the mud. Stir the mud occasionally.

2 Cut a piece of highly porous cloth (such as cheesecloth or heavy gauze) into a 12-by-12-inch square. Lay it unfolded on a heat-resistant surface. When the mud has heated thoroughly, take the smaller bowl out of the hot water. With a spatula, scoop all the mud out of the bowl onto the center of the cloth. Mound the mud so that it's about an inch or two thick in the center. Fold each corner of the cloth on top of the mud to form a neat pack.

3 Position the mud pack directly on any area of your body causing you discomfort. Be sure to keep the folded layers of cloth on top, and the thin, porous layer against your skin. Wind some plastic wrap around the affected area to retain the heat, then cover it with a towel. Leave the pack on for 20 to 30 minutes.

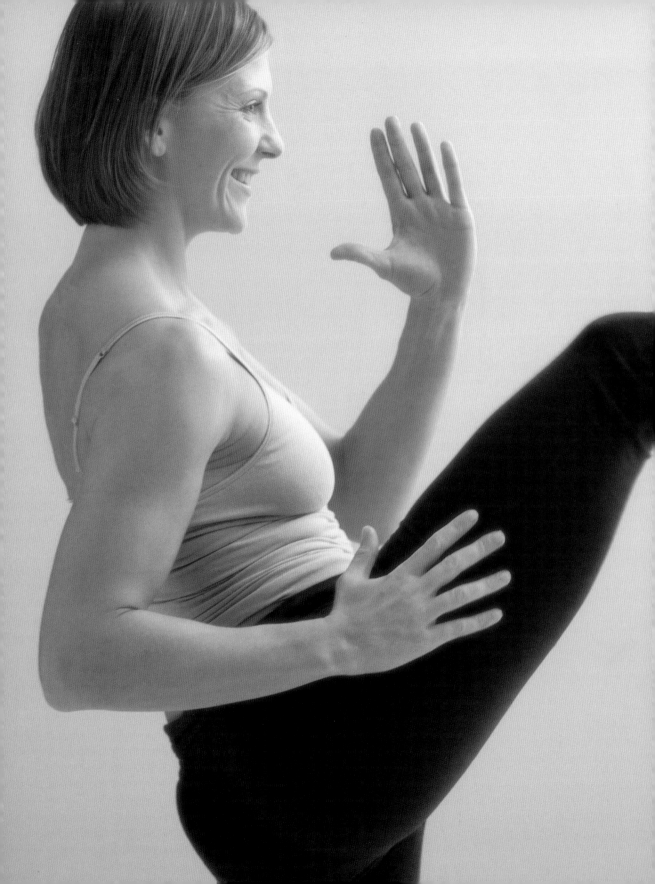

People all over the world have been using sweat to cleanse their bodies—and even purify their souls—for centuries. The Finnish have their hutlike saunas. The Russians enjoy the cavernous public baths known as *banyas*. The Japanese *sentos* offer a variety of bathing options (including hot and cold pools), and the Native Americans build sweat lodges heated with hot rocks to rid their bodies and minds of impurities, and to commune with the spirits.

working up a sweat

Sweat—a mixture of water, sodium chloride, potassium salts, urea, and lactic acid—cools the body via evaporation. Whether or not sweat actually flushes out environmental toxins is up for debate, but getting hot enough to make your body sweat is certainly healthy: It improves blood circulation, helps rid the body of normal waste products, loosens muscles, and gives you rosy cheeks. Equally important, a good sweating session makes you feel better: cleaner, more relaxed, and profoundly renewed.

You may not have a sauna or steam bath at your disposal, but that doesn't mean you need to forgo the pleasures of perspiration. Vigorous exercise—whether it's a kickboxing class, a long run, or chasing your kids around a playground—can also help you work up a good sweat. In some cultures and eras, women weren't supposed to sweat, as it was considered unfeminine. Today, active women believe in physical strength and vigor, and they know that it's healthy—even a sign of power—to break into a sweat.

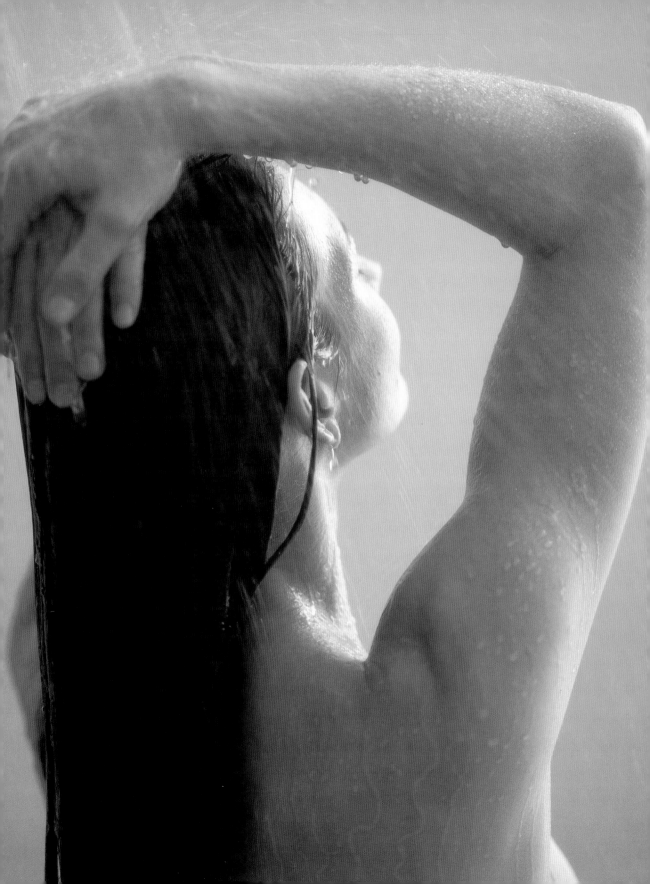

hangover relief

When you've partied a little too hearty, only time will completely clear your head and settle your stomach. But some simple detox techniques speed the process along.

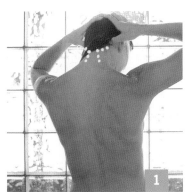 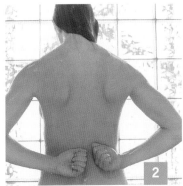 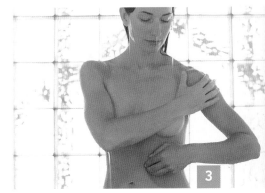

1 To help relieve nausea and headaches, press your thumbs into the muscles and acupressure points along your skull and neck. Start by placing your thumbs at the base of your skull, one on each side of the upper spine. Press in for two breaths, release, and move an inch outward; repeat until you're an inch or so away from your ears. Return to the upper spine and press on each side again, inching your thumbs down your neck until you reach the top of the shoulders.

2 Lend your detoxification filters a hand by gently pummeling your kidneys, helping to break up toxic crystal deposits. Leaning over slightly, reach behind you and, with soft fists, gently pound below your lower ribs, about 12 times on each side, using comfortable pressure.

3 The acupressure point known as Spleen 16 is a classic target for relief from hangover symptoms. Using the fingertips of one hand, find the bottom of your rib cage and move your hand directly in line with your nipple. Feel for a slight indentation in the bone, and then press gently upward into the ribs. Hold the point for a count of ten full breaths. Repeat on the other side.

Relief Reinforcements

A few more hangover tips: Drink plenty of water to rehydrate your body; adding a little lemon juice helps the detoxification effect. Resuscitate yourself with a cool compress on which you've sprinkled three drops of lavender, peppermint, or rosemary essential oil. If you're nauseous, use rose or sandalwood oil instead. And take a vitamin B supplement—granted, this is more effective if taken right before your binge, but it will still help you feel better the next morning.

part the horse's mane

With its flowing, continual movements, tai chi stimulates the circulation of blood and lymphatic fluid, aiding the body's natural detoxification mechanisms.

1 Looking over your left shoulder and keeping your feet close together, bend your left knee and raise your heel so the toes of your left foot rest gently on the ground. Hold your arms out in a rounded position, as if you're holding a large ball, with your palms facing each other. Your left hand should be down by your waist; your right arm should be raised to about shoulder height.

2 Step out with your left leg so that you land on your left heel, toes pointing up. Keeping your head, back, and buttocks in a straight line, sweep your arms past each other, moving your left hand out and up and your right hand out and down, with the palms facing each other.

3 Firmly plant your left foot. Bend the knee so it's in line with your toes. Keep your right leg extended. Extend your left hand to a little lower than shoulder height, with the elbow gently bent and the palm facing you. Move your right hand down by your waist, with a slight bend at the elbow and your palm facing down. Now repeat the movements on the other side, and then alternate both sides again.

KEEPING BODY FLUIDS IN BALANCE

As blood circulates, it carries oxygen, glucose, proteins, and other nutrients throughout your body. Some of these essential components are lost, however, when plasma leaks through the walls of blood vessels and gets trapped in tissue cells. The lymphatic system drains away the trapped fluid and nutrients, along with waste products and germs, and deposits them back into the bloodstream. This system is powered by the pumping of the muscles surrounding the lymphatic vessels; massaging the pathways helps promote this vital activity.

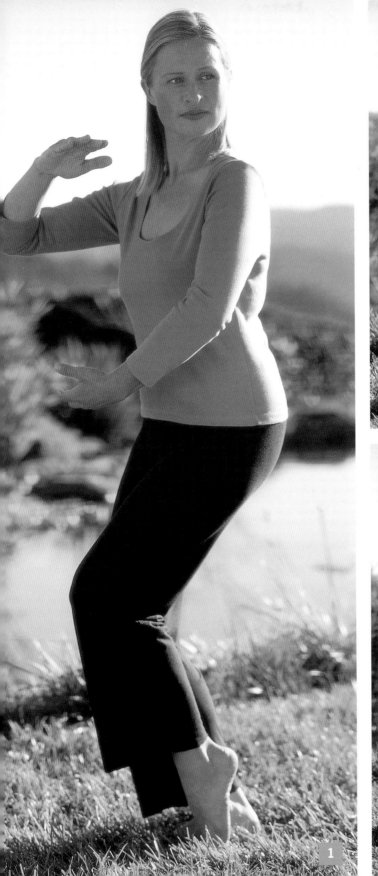

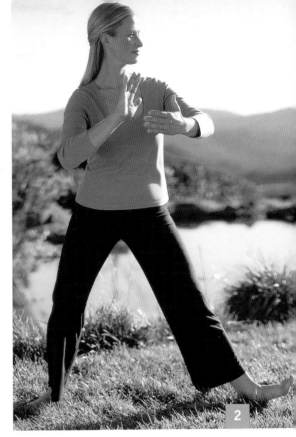

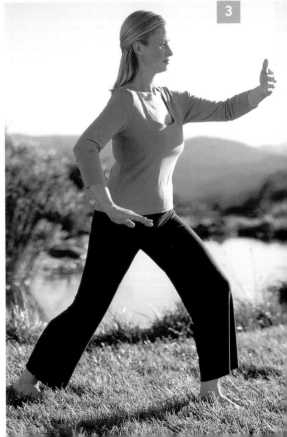

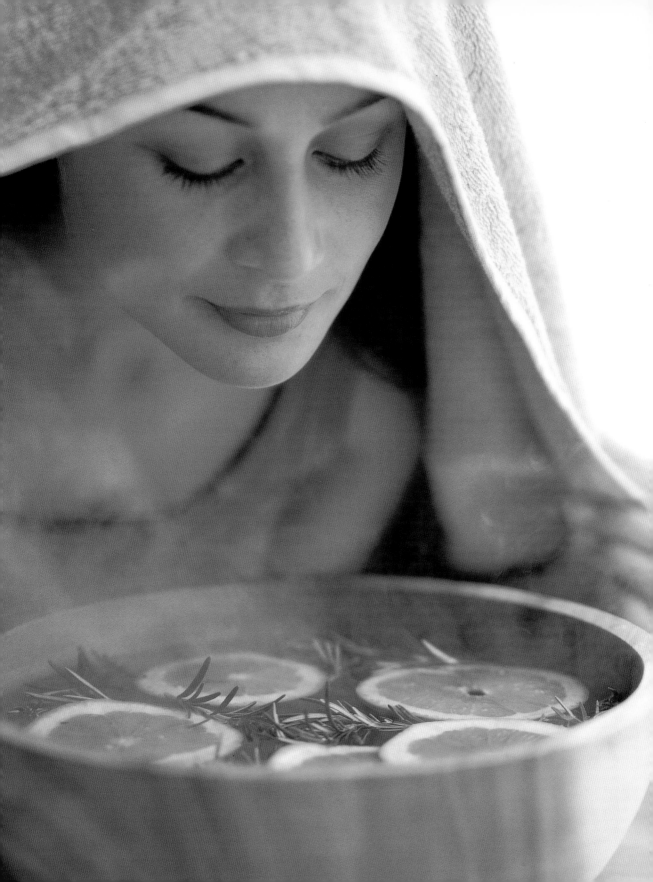

essential steam

Steam treatments help release toxins stored in the fatty tissue just under the skin. Adding certain aromatic oils to the steam can intensify the detoxifying effect.

Fill a bowl with boiling water. Add grapefruit and rosemary essential oils (see recipe at right), as well as sprigs of fresh rosemary and slices of grapefruit if desired. Lean over the bowl, taking care to keep your face about 12 inches away. Let comfort be your guide—this should be a pleasant experience, not an endurance test. Drape a bath towel over your head and the bowl to trap the vapors. (If the vapors sting your eyes, keep them closed.) Steam your face for five to ten minutes.

If you're not especially fond of grapefruit and rosemary, many other essential oils, including juniper, geranium, Atlas cedar, sweet orange, and bay laurel, also offer helpful detoxifying benefits. Experiment with individual oils and then try blends of oils to discover which seem most pleasing and effective to you.

After you've completed your treatment, remember that steamed skin is fragile. Gently apply a moisturizer appropriate for your skin type (see page 57 ◄) while your face is still slightly damp from the steaming. Top off your steam by drinking water or a dandelion tonic (see page 120 ►); either will help flush out the released toxins.

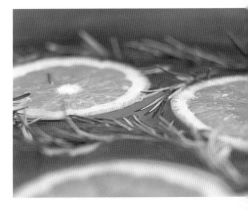

Detoxifying Steam Blend

Large bowl filled with boiling water

3 drops grapefruit essential oil

2 drops rosemary essential oil

4 sprigs fresh rosemary (optional)

4 grapefruit slices (optional)

Bath towel

THE VIRTUES OF GETTING ALL STEAMED UP

Besides coaxing your body to release toxins, steaming opens up the skin's pores, helping to dislodge any grime and make-up residue, and imparts vital moisture to deeper skin layers. It softens dead skin cells, making it easier to exfoliate them with a gentle facial scrub, and can make blackheads easier to remove. A good steaming session also increases circulation to your face and relaxes facial muscles, both of which contribute to a refreshed, pleasing glow.

Skin-Savvy Ingredients

Aromatherapists often recommend grapefruit essential oil to relieve acne and tone the skin. You can use it in a steam blend, as shown, or add it to a base lotion to create a healing moisturizer. Rosemary oil also serves as an astringent and an antibacterial agent that helps prevent pimples.

half spinal twist

While yoga poses cultivate flexibility and strength, they also can provide compression that massages the internal organs, helping to cleanse the body of toxins.

Easy and rewarding even for beginners, this twisting pose helps massage and tone the liver, spleen, and intestines, which yogis say makes Half Spinal Twist ideal for detoxification purposes.

Sitting on the ground, place your right foot on the left side of your left calf. Your left leg will be straight on the ground; your right knee will be bent. Sit up straight and inhale as you elongate your spine.

Exhale as you turn toward your right, rotating from the base of your spine upward. Bring your right hand to the ground behind your back for support, and place your left arm on the right side of your leg to increase your leverage as you twist as far as you comfortably can.

Look over your right shoulder. Hold for 30 seconds while continuing to twist gently and breathe deeply. On an exhale, untwist slowly. Turn your head forward and release from your shoulders downward as you bring your body back to center. Repeat on your left side. (If your back feels a little tight, see page 130 ▶ for back-soothing yoga poses.)

DETOXING THE MIND

Anyone who has taken a yoga class knows it can clean your mind of stress and mental clutter. But yoga is good for more than just temporary relief of emotional toxins. German researchers found that women who practiced yoga showed markedly higher scores in life satisfaction than a control group (who simply read books), as well as lower scores in excitability, aggressiveness, emotionality, and physical complaints. Those in the yogi group also coped better with stress and were cheerier and more extroverted.

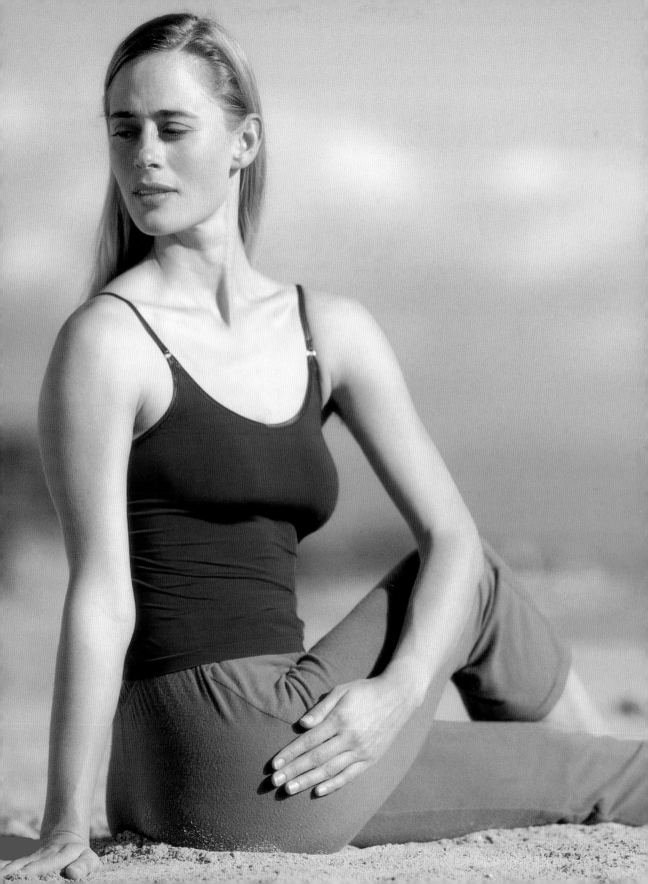

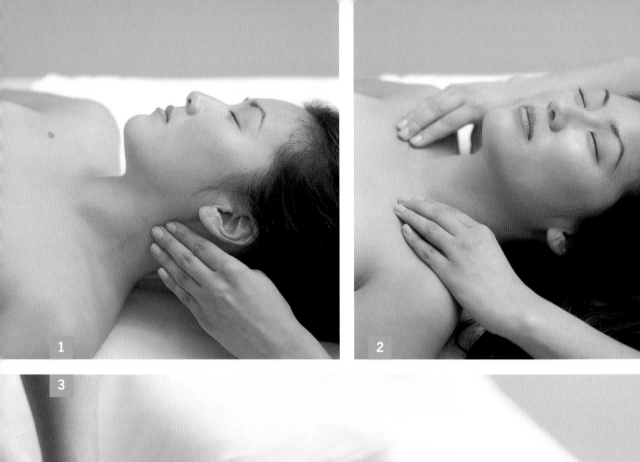

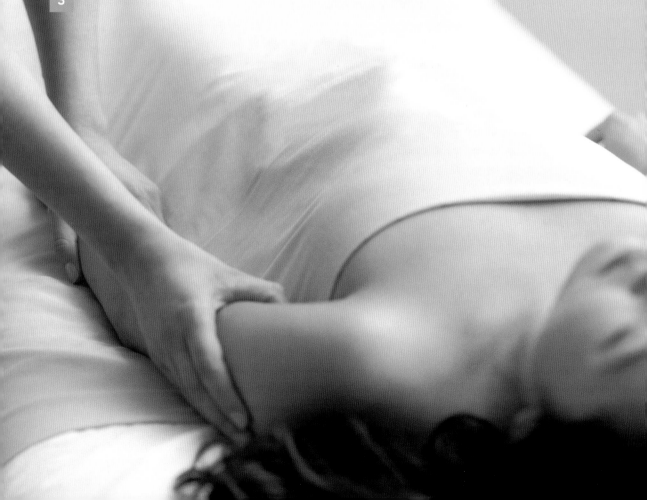

purifying massage

Massage is a powerful weapon in the detox arsenal.
Firm and targeted manipulation improves circulation and
helps flush out chemical deposits trapped in muscles.

Too much exercise, stress, or alcohol use, as well as poor dietary
habits, can leave irritating chemical deposits locked between muscle
fibers, causing discomfort and making the muscles sluggish. Flushing
out these chemicals helps alleviate pain and creates healthier muscles
that respond better and have more stamina. The deep gliding strokes
in this massage have a sweeping effect on the fluids of the body and
also help propel blood briskly back toward the heart and lungs, where
it feasts on oxygen before making another trip through the body. Ask
a friend to follow these massage steps to help you detox:

1 Pour a little room-temperature massage oil in your hands (see the
recipe at right if you want to use a home-brewed blend with essential
oils). Starting an inch or so below the ear on the thick muscles at the
side of the neck, use the pads of your fingers to glide lightly down
the sides of her neck, angling in toward the breastbone.

2 With flat fingers on top of the breastbone, sweep out across the
chest muscles to the front of the shoulders. Sweep your hands back
around and under the shoulder muscles and press firmly toward the
base of her neck. Glide up the muscles along each side of the spine
in the neck to the base of the skull. Repeat Steps 1 and 2 five times.

3 Stabilize one of her forearms with one hand, and wrap the fingers
and thumb of your other hand around her forearm. Press in and glide
up to the shoulder. Curve around the shoulder and glide lightly back
down her arm. Do this five times and then repeat on the other arm.
Move to her legs and position your hands so they overlap and wrap
around one of her ankles. Then press in with your fingers and thumbs
and lightly glide up to the knee. Lighten the pressure more as you
move over the knee itself, then glide from knee to hip and back
down to the ankle. Repeat five times, then massage the other leg.

Detoxifying Massage Oil Blend

2 ounces carrier oil of choice

8 drops cypress essential oil

8 drops juniper essential oil

5 drops lavender essential oil

4 drops orange essential oil

Toxins, Toxins Everywhere…
Proponents of detox therapies claim
that external toxins come from such
sources as overly processed foods,
pollution, and clothing made of
artificial fibers. (Our bodies also
make their own toxic stew in the
form of normal waste products.)
To combat these contaminants, detox
advocates recommend regimens
ranging from juice fasts to colonics.
It's always best to consult with a
doctor before trying such methods.

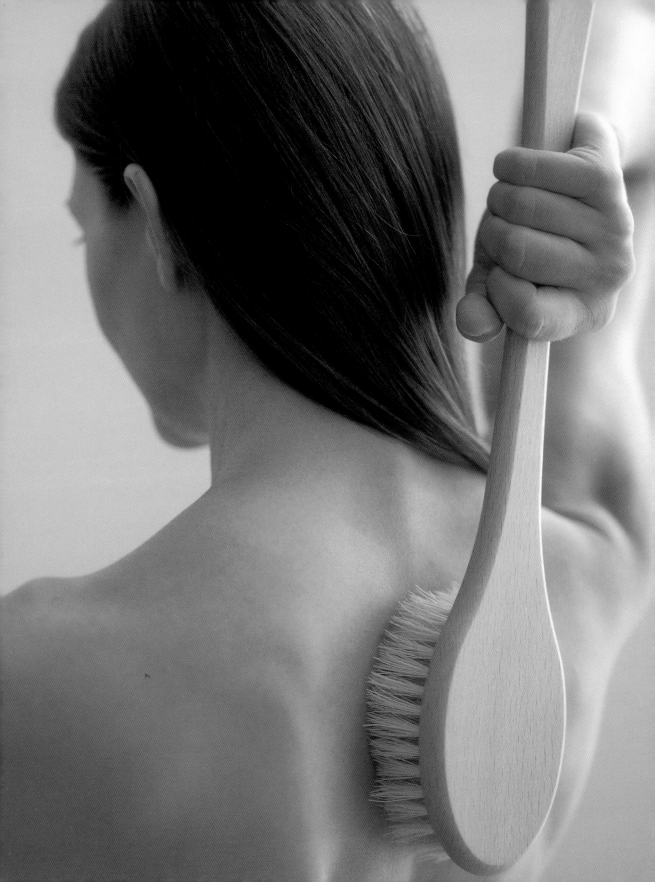

dry body brushing

Popular in European spas, this treatment exfoliates dead skin cells, gets blood circulating, and helps stimulate the lymphatic system. It's also easy to do daily.

Using a long-handled brush with soft, natural bristles, start brushing your back. Apply light pressure and brush everywhere you can comfortably reach. Then gently brush your legs, arms, shoulders, abdomen, and buttocks. When brushing to stimulate the lymphatic system, always brush toward your heart (that is, downward when working on your shoulders or upper back, upward when working on your limbs). The whole routine should take only a few minutes; then you're ready to jump into the shower.

Once in the shower, you can intensify the stimulating effect of the treatment by fluctuating the temperature of the water. After you've finished washing with soap and rinsing off your body, decrease the temperature of the shower and rinse with cold water for about 15 seconds. Then adjust the temperature of the water back up to warm for a minute or so. End your shower with a five-second blast of cold water. The temperature changes in the water will exercise capillary walls and tone tissues, encouraging better circulation.

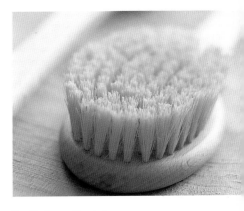

The Basics on Brushes

The best dry body brushes use natural fibers, cactus, or Japanese palm. Many brushes have long handles for hard-to-reach places. Warning: Never use a body brush on varicose veins, or if you have eczema, psoriasis, or other skin irritations.

GIVING CELLULITE THE BRUSH-OFF

The cellulite that collects on most women's thighs and buttocks occurs when collagen fibrils, irritated by the buildup of toxins, wrap themselves around fat cells, sealing in the fat and toxins. The result? A lumpy, orange-peel look. Other factors, such as sluggish blood circulation and insufficient lymphatic drainage, exacerbate the problem. Dry body brushing helps by stimulating the circulatory system and encouraging the flow of lymphatic fluid. Following up with a knobby massage glove encourages collagen fibrils to soften and mobilizes fat cells, so they can be flushed out of your body.

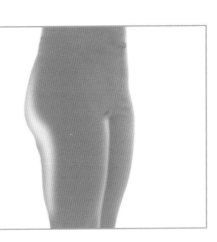

detox

dandelion tonic

The common dandelion turns out to be uncommonly rich in vitamins and nutrients. Here it joins forces with other healthy ingredients to create a detoxifying tonic.

Ingredients

2 tablespoons tender green
 celery leaves

1 tablespoon fresh Italian parsley

8 mint leaves

6 ounces pineapple juice

15 to 20 drops dandelion root tincture

2 to 3 drops Tabasco green
 jalapeño sauce

Celery stalk or fresh, whole
 strawberry (optional)

• Serves: 1 (¾-cup serving)

• Prep time: 10 minutes

Nutritional Information Per Serving

This tonic's many virtues include being fat- and cholesterol-free.

Calories	110
Kilojoules	440
Protein	1 g
Carbohydrates	26 g
Total Fat	0 g
Saturated Fat	0 g
Cholesterol	0 mg
Sodium	20 mg
Dietary Fiber	0 g

Who would have thought that the humble dandelion, that bane of lawn-proud homeowners, would prove to be a nutritional bonanza and a highly effective detoxification agent? But it's true: Dandelions contain more vitamin A than carrots, more vitamin C than tomatoes, as much iron as spinach, and more potassium than bananas. They also help rid the body of excess fluids and waste materials—without draining the supply of potassium, as many other diuretics do.

If you need a little detoxing, try this tasty tonic. The dandelion root tincture (sold at health food stores) will help, and the pineapple has its own detoxifying qualities. This tonic also is rich in vitamins A, B, and C, as well as bromelain, an enzyme that helps digest protein.

1 Chop the celery leaves, Italian parsley, and mint leaves and place them in a blender. Add the pineapple juice, dandelion root tincture, and jalapeño sauce. Blend on high speed until thoroughly mixed.

2 Pour through a coarse sieve into a glass filled with ice. Garnish with a celery stalk or fresh strawberry, and serve immediately.

WEED IT AND REAP

The dandelion has long been lauded for its culinary and medicinal value. Dandelions were used by the ancient Egyptians to alleviate stomach and kidney ailments, ranked among the original bitter herbs used in the Jewish Passover, and gained much favor among 16th-century English aristocrats as a cure-all. Traditional healers use it to treat ailments ranging from constipation to eczema. Every part is edible, from the roots, which can be roasted, to the greens, which add zing to salads, to the flowers, which are used to make wine.

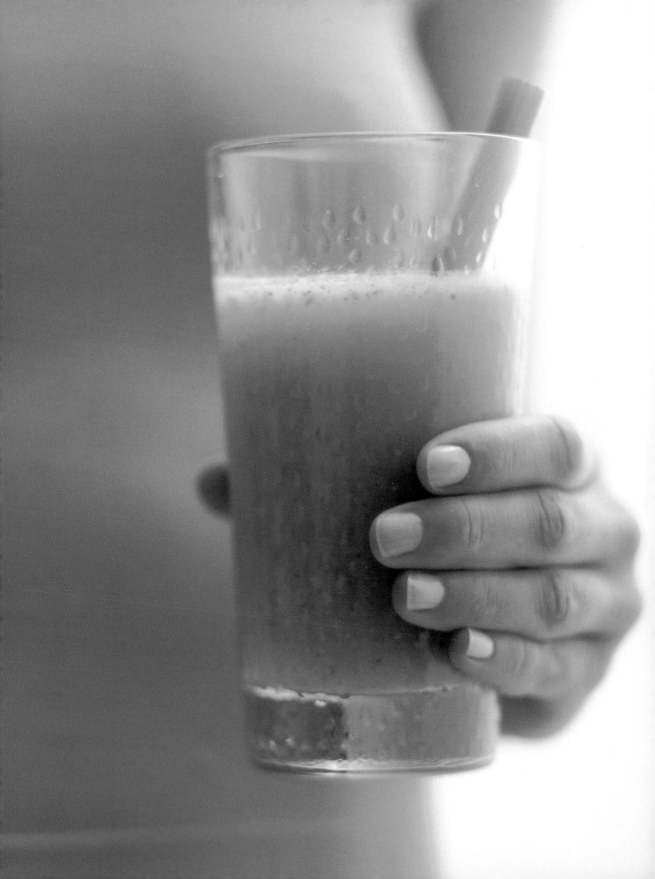

relieve

Your muscles ache, your eyes are tired, your mind feels clouded with fatigue. You can reach into the medicine cabinet for an antidote, or you can try some of these pure and simple self-help remedies.

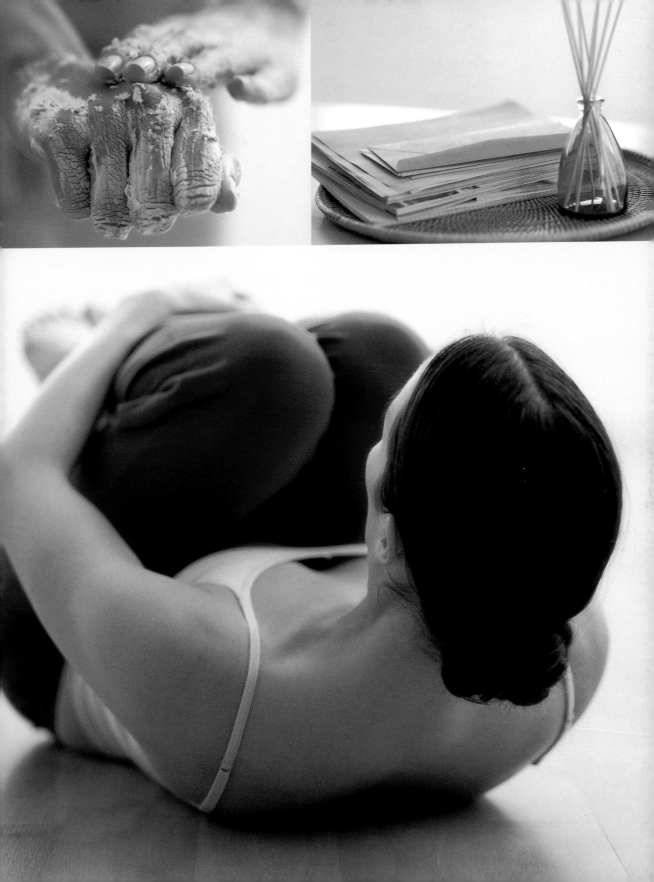

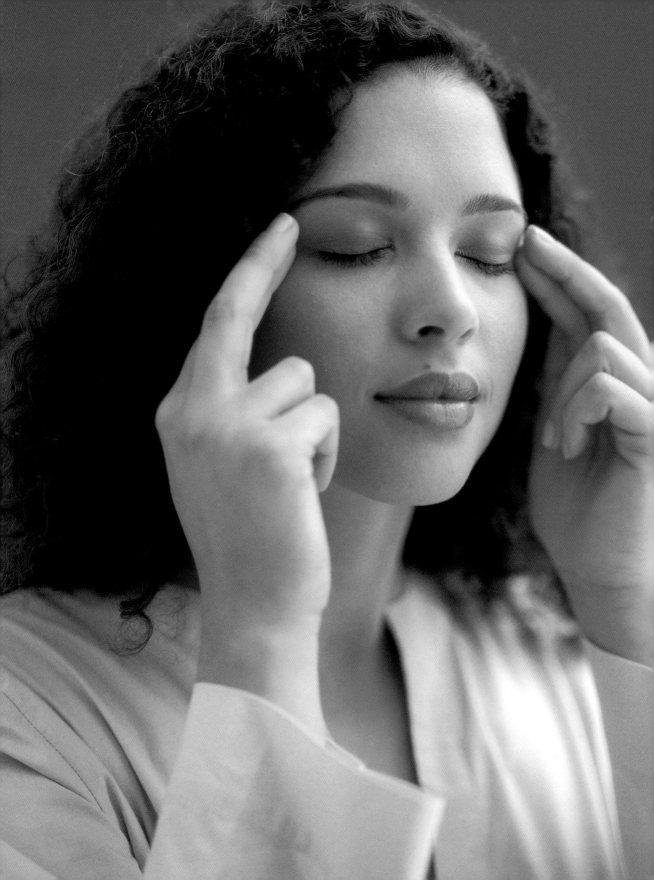

relieve

Whether you're working, in school, or staying at home with the kids, your daily routines—never mind those spur-of-the-moment crises—can wreak havoc on your mind and body. Studies show that about 80 percent of the world's population suffers from back pain at some point, and nearly the same percentage is plagued with frequent headaches. Add to that common maladies such as eyestrain, sore feet, tight muscles, and the yearly dose of colds and flus, and you get the picture: Life isn't always easy.

Pain-killing pills, magical lotions, and expensive potions all promise ready relief from the ills that come with modern living. Sometimes what's needed, though, is a simpler (but no less potent) cure: a steaming bowl of chicken soup to ease the misery of a cold, a yoga pose to help relax tight back muscles, a soothing touch applied to aching calf muscles or bleary eyes. You'll find many such remedies and activities on the following pages, and all are easy to do and have been proven safe and effective. As you contemplate which of the treatments might best suit your needs, keep in mind that your general attitude is equally important: that making time for a healthy dose of self-care is a necessity, not an indulgence.

relieve

sports massage for arms

Self-massage using compression, cross-fiber friction, and direct pressure can help you warm up before a workout and soothe joint or muscle pain afterward.

When Good Fibers Go Bad
Skeletal muscle fibers run parallel to one another, sliding against each other thousands of times a day as they relax and contract with every movement. Stress, poor diet, insufficient fluids, bad posture, fatigue, overuse, and a host of other factors can cause these fibers to stick together, making you feel stiff and sore in places. Rolling your thumb, fingers, knuckles, or elbows across the grain of the muscles starts to separate the fibers, releasing the chemical glue that binds them.

1 With one hand braced on the back of your head, sink your fingertips into the front edge of your armpit to position them under your chest muscles. Squeeze your thumb and fingers together. Work the length of the muscle from top to bottom, squeezing and rolling across the ropey muscle fibers. Repeat three times (or until you feel the muscles relax), and then work on the other arm.

2 Increase circulation and release the tension in your biceps with compression. Rest your elbow on your knee or on a table. With your palm flat against the inside of your biceps just above your elbow and your fingers wrapped around your arm, squeeze firmly, then release. Rhythmically pump in this manner as you move from elbow to shoulder. Do three times; then repeat on the other arm.

3 To help relieve forearm tension, sink the fingers of one hand into the muscles on the top of your opposite forearm and firmly rub across the muscles from side to side, feeling them roll under the pressure (this is what's known as cross-fiber friction). Work them for three to five seconds. Release your grip slightly and repeat the move as you make your way from elbow to wrist. When you've covered the length of your forearm, repeat on the other arm.

4 If any areas on your arms are sore, soothe them with direct pressure. Take a deep breath, and as you exhale, press your thumb slowly into a sore spot. The pressure should be firm, but not enough to cause acute discomfort. Breathe normally and hold the point for 10 to 30 seconds before releasing the pressure gradually. Press, hold, and release three times on each sore spot. (Now that your arms are primed, try the strengthening exercises on page 87 ◄.)

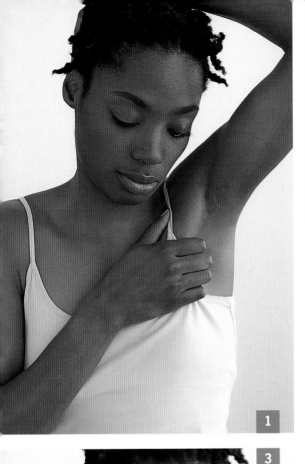

1

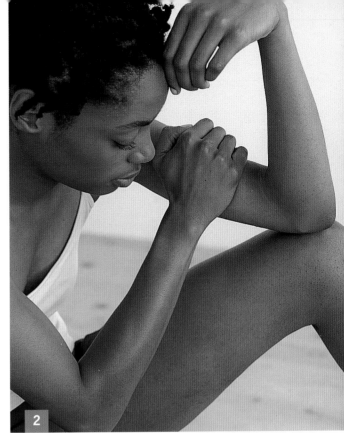

2

3

4

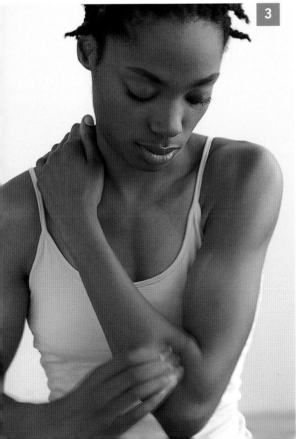

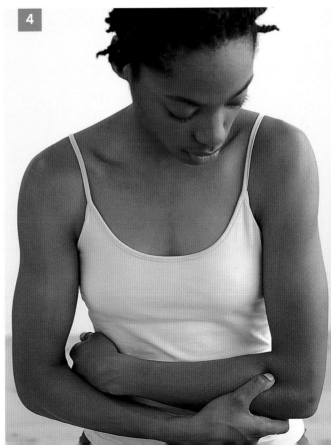

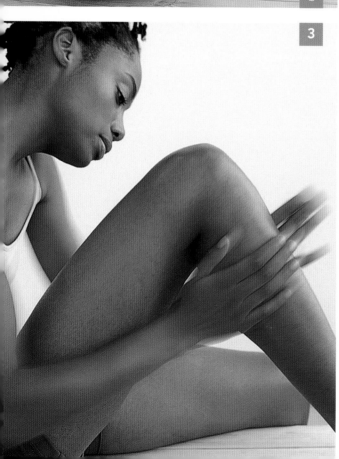

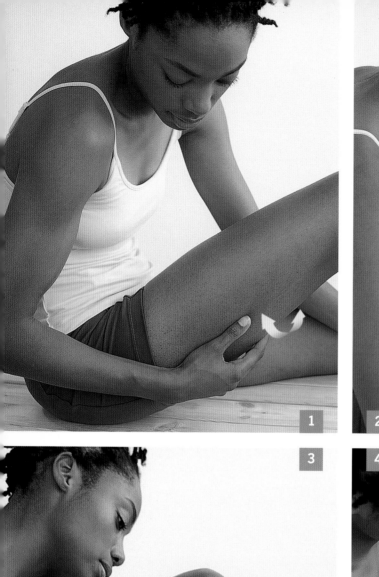

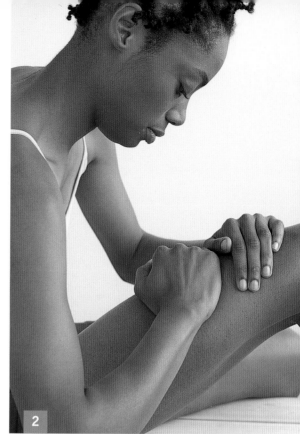

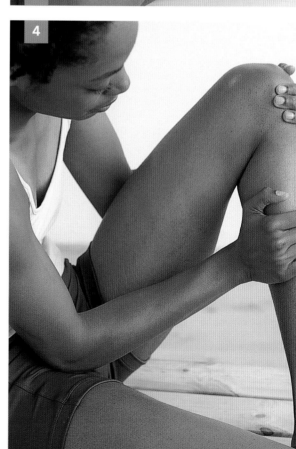

1

2

3

4

sports massage for legs

Just like stretching before and after workouts, these easy and effective self-massage techniques will help warm you up, pump you up, and even undo damage.

1 Tight hamstrings slow you down, decrease leg power, and make you wear out more quickly. Relax tension by giving your leg muscles a little jiggle before beginning to exercise. Sit on the ground or a bench, bend one knee up slightly, and grasp the muscles on the underside of that thigh with one hand. Begin waggling them loosely from side to side. Move up and down the length of your thigh, jostling your leg muscles as you go. Switch hands if one tires. Do six times, and then repeat on the other leg.

2 Exercise can cause a painful buildup of lactic acid and metabolic wastes in your muscles. Help flush out these unwanted deposits from your thighs by compressing your quadriceps. Sit on the ground or a bench and bend one knee up slightly, as before. With the heels of both palms, press down into your thigh muscles, squeezing toward the bone in a pumping action. Release the pressure and move to a new spot, repeating from knee to hip. For extra power, rock your body forward as you press in, and lean back on your release. Work both of your legs from the knee to the hip six times.

3 To help move toxins and waste out of your calf, roll the muscles. With palms pressed into the fleshy part of your calf, rapidly push up with one hand while pulling down with the other, creating a rolling motion, for 30 seconds. Work both of your legs.

4 Relieve fluid congestion and soreness in your calves with compression. Starting near one ankle, press with the heel of your palm straight in toward the bone, and release. Pump the calf muscles in a rhythmic manner, moving toward your knee. Repeat this set of compressions three times, then work the other leg. (Your legs now should be ready to take on the strengthening exercises on page 88 ◂.)

Heat It Up or Cool It Down?

Most sports injuries are sprains (damage to ligaments, which link bones together), strains (damage to tendons, which bind muscles to bones), and contusions (bruises). In most cases, medical professionals recommend treating such injuries with RICE: Rest (don't exercise the injured body part), Ice (ten to 30 minutes, several times a day, for a day or two), Compress (with an elastic cloth bandage), and Elevate (keep the injured part above your heart). After the swelling goes down, applying heat can help to alleviate any remaining discomfort.

back soothers

Regular yoga practice increases the range of motion in your back and hips, massages your abdominal organs, and stretches and strengthens core muscles.

Our Aching Backs
In the United States, lower back pain is the most common cause of missed workdays, the leading cause of disability in people aged 19 to 45, and the most common complaint of *all* medical patients. In fact, doctors expect some 80 percent of the world's population to suffer from back pain at some point in their lives. What's to blame? Sedentary lifestyles, poor posture, too much time on unsupportive mattresses and in poorly fitted chairs, and carrying heavy loads have all contributed to what seems to be an international epidemic of back pain.

1 The pelvic tilt feels good on its own, and it also is used in many *asanas* (yoga poses)—as well as other forms of exercise—to protect the lower back from strain. To assume this soothing pose, lie on your back on a comfortable surface with your knees bent and your feet on the floor hip-width apart. Your arms should rest on the floor alongside your body. Inhale, arching your lower back and pressing your tailbone down. Then exhale, flattening your lower back down to the floor and pressing your tailbone upward. Continue this pattern for four to ten breaths, arching your back with each inhalation and then flattening your back with each exhalation.

2 Still lying on your back, bring your legs together with your knees bent and extend your arms out from your shoulders along the floor, with your palms down. Lower your bent legs toward the floor to your left, keeping your right shoulder grounded. Gaze either upward or, if you can do so comfortably, to your right. If you like, you can hold your left hand on your knees to add a little more weight on your legs. Hold for ten breaths, and inhale as you bring your legs back to center, then repeat on your right side.

3 Now, lying on your back, bring your knees to your chest and wrap your arms around your legs. Inhale deeply and hold your breath as you lift your chest toward your knees. Then rock, either from side to side or from head to hips, using the weight of your body to massage your back. When you're ready to exhale, release your breath all at once through your mouth and, at the same time, stretch out your limbs on the floor. Relax for a minute or two, then repeat. (Half Spinal Twist also stretches the back; see page 114 ◄.)

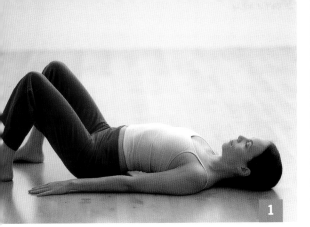

1

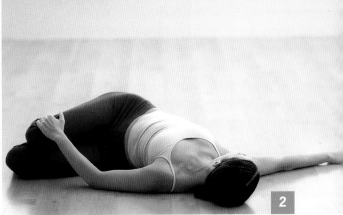

2

3

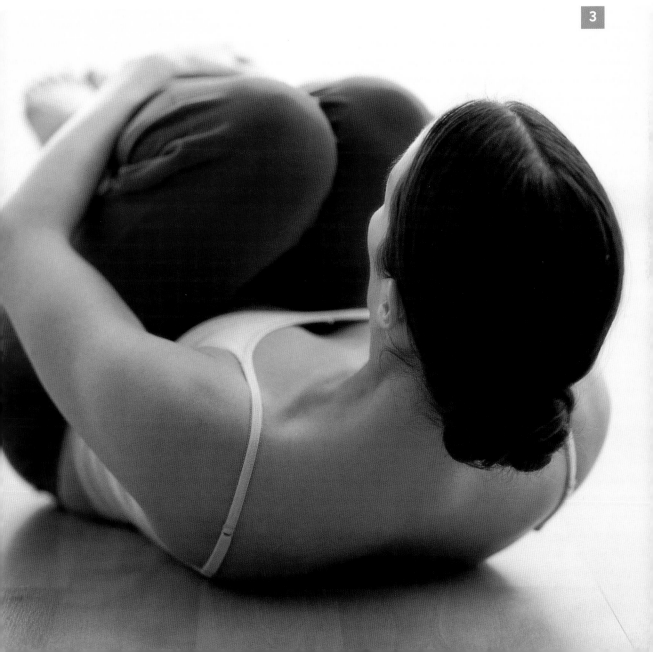

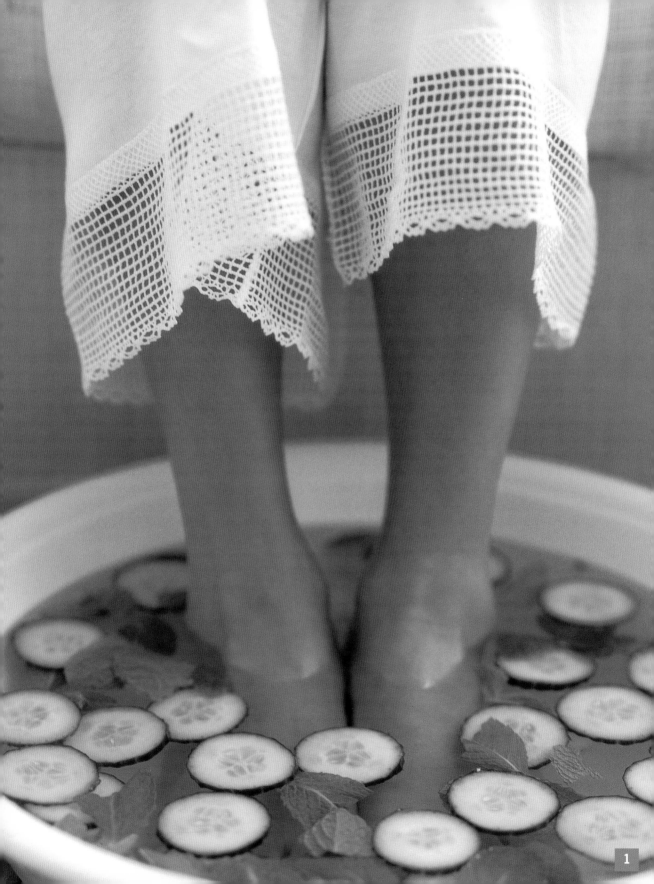

time-out for tired feet

When your feet are weary and ache after a long day, soak, roll, and massage your way to immediate relief with this trio of soothing at-home spa treatments.

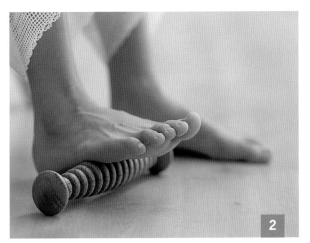

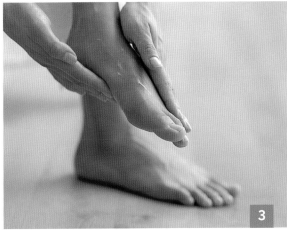

1 Fill a large bowl with cool water. Add six drops of tea tree essential oil and stir. Then add a couple dozen cucumber slices and a handful of torn fresh mint leaves. (Tea tree oil has antibacterial properties, cucumber acts as a mild astringent, and mint imparts a fresh scent.) Place the bowl at the foot of your favorite chair and ease your feet into the water. Relax, and soak your feet for about 15 minutes.

2 After your soak, sit comfortably in a chair, place one foot on a wooden foot roller, and move it forward and back, varying the speed and pressure. Massage for five to ten minutes, then switch feet.

3 Give your feet a manual massage. Using a generous amount of lotion, balm, or massage oil with an appealing scent, vigorously massage one foot, rubbing briskly back and forth. Then, with your hands wrapped around the arch of your foot, squeeze your hands together firmly and glide them toward your toes. This action increases circulation and helps remove toxins. Repeat on your other foot.

Rolling for Reflexology

When you use a wooden foot roller, you're actually doing much more than simply soothing your aching feet: The foot roller is designed to activate the reflexology zones of the soles of your feet (see page 201 ▶). You can easily avail yourself of this refreshing action by keeping a wooden roller—or even a few golf balls placed in a sock—around for a quickie foot massage during the day.

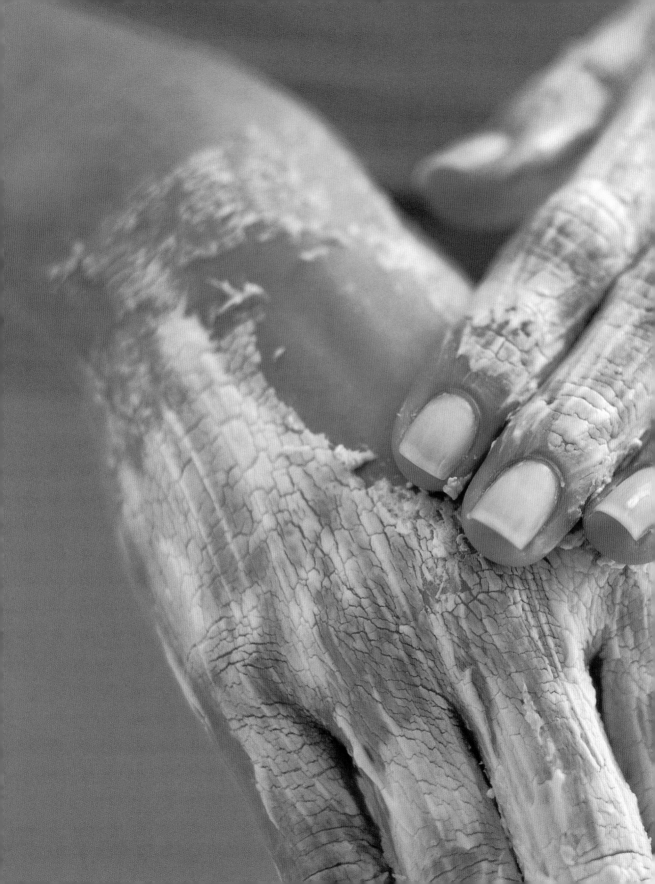

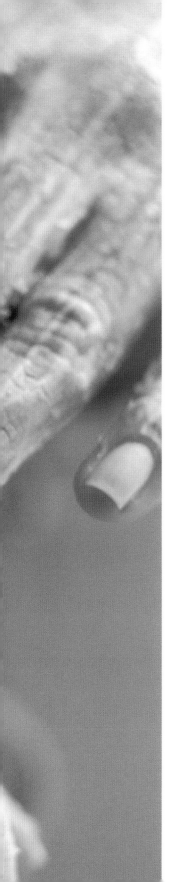

sweet almond oil

Give your hands a well-deserved scrub with products featuring sweet almond oil, a light and delicately scented oil that promotes soft skin and flexible nails.

The human hand is capable of myriad gestures and tasks—from caressing a lover's face to grasping a child's hand, from tooling a piece of leather to washing endless dishes, from simply waving good-bye to communicating in sign language. We often forget how hard our hands work until we notice they are sore, rough, or heavily lined.

Pampering your hands from time to time makes them look and feel better, and a complete treatment involves more than just getting your nails done. Instead, try exfoliating, conditioning, and moisturizing your hands with a trio of sweet almond oil products. A key ingredient in many massage and moisturizing lotions, sweet almond oil is ideal for dry, chapped, mature, or simply overworked hands because it contains essential fatty acids, which protect and replenish the skin and help keep nails healthy and supple.

To intensify the effects of this moisturizing process, slip on a pair of hand-treatment gloves (or clean socks). Leave them on for a few minutes, or even overnight if your hands are particularly dry.

NOT REALLY A NUT

Neither nut nor legume, the sweet almond (the formal name for the common snack food) is actually a fruit. Most of us never see the flesh of that fruit; hard, leathery, and dull green, it dries up when ripe, leaving a rough shell in which lies the actual kernel that we eat and use for oil. In addition to its virtues as a beauty aid, almond oil is an excellent salad and cooking oil: It is light tasting, has the benefit of being cholesterol free, and has a high flash point (which means that it doesn't burn easily).

step-by-step sequence ▶

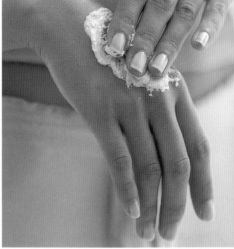

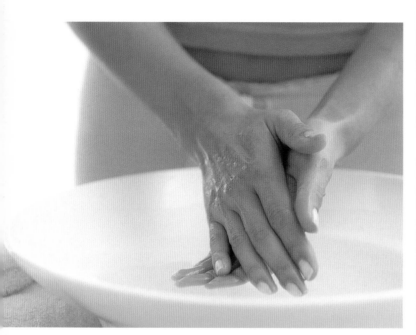

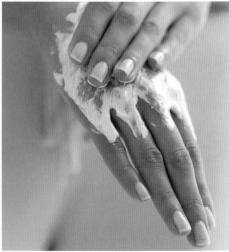

1 Fill a bowl or sink with warm water and wash your hands with a mild soap. Avoid using very hot water, as it can further dry your skin. Wash your hands slowly and purposefully. Take a few minutes to massage them by pressing your thumbs into your palms, and gently squeeze each finger, working from the bottom to the top of each. Then rinse and dry your hands.

2 Once your hands are completely dry, spread an exfoliating scrub containing sweet almond oil on the back of each hand. Put a thick, even layer of the scrub on your hands and over the entire length of your fingers. Then allow the scrub to dry for about ten minutes.

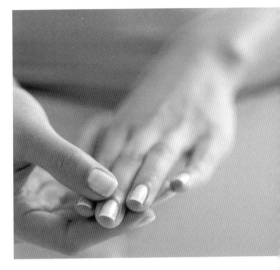

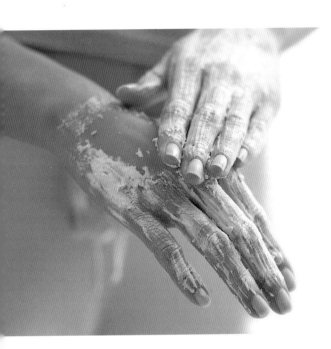

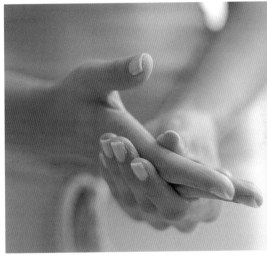

3 When the scrub has a chalky consistency, you'll know it's dry and ready to remove. Simply rub your hands together until most of the product flakes off. Or use a clean, dry washcloth to thoroughly brush the scrub off your hands.

4 Now condition your nails and cuticles with sweet almond oil nail balm. Massage a generous amount onto the surface of each nail and into the cuticle. When the nail balm has been absorbed, finish by applying a highly emollient sweet almond cream liberally over both hands.

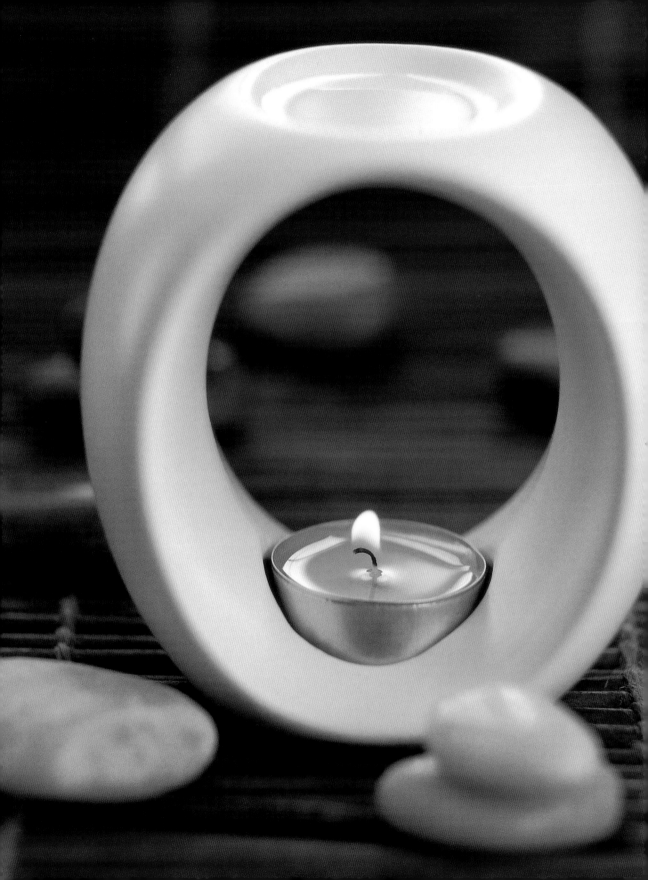

aromatherapy diffusers

When you're feeling stressed, anxious, or sad, help brighten your mood by infusing your environment with the soothing aroma of uplifting essential oils.

Dispersing pure essential oils in a diffuser to release their aromas is a pleasing and effective way to create a mood and unleash their various therapeutic properties. Many types of aromatherapy diffusers now are available—clay, glass, ceramic, and metal—and some are as decorative as they are efficient. They are designed with dishes or wells in which to place the essential oils, which are usually diluted with water or a carrier oil (follow the manufacturer's instructions on the proper use of your particular model). Many are warmed by small candles, but electric diffusers that circulate cool air are gaining in popularity. If you use candles in your diffuser, make sure they're unscented, so they don't interfere with the aroma produced by the oils you've selected.

To help relieve tension, anxiety, or sadness, try diffusing oils such as ylang-ylang, lavender, and rose. Neroli, bergamot, geranium, clary sage, and palma rosa are also considered calming and help restore a sense of balance and optimism—a useful air freshener, indeed.

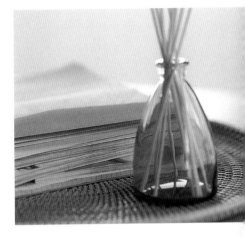

Reed Diffusers
A reed diffuser—in which an essential oil travels up a series of slender bamboo reeds—allows you to have an ongoing release of beneficial aromas in your home or office without the drawbacks of some other kinds of diffusers. For example, the reed diffuser doesn't require electricity or use a candle, thus removing the risk of fire.

FLOWER POWER

To date, few scientific studies have been undertaken to test the effectiveness of aromatherapy. However, some do back up claims that certain essential oils relieve stress and anxiety. Researchers at the Sloan-Kettering Cancer Center in New York found that the scent of heliotrope helped patients relax during MRI scans. In another study, patients who received foot rubs with neroli essential oil after undergoing heart surgery exhibited less anxiety than those patients massaged with unscented oil. In Scotland, researchers found that rubbing a solution containing thyme, rosemary, lavender, and cedar essential oils onto the scalps of patients suffering from *alopecia areata*, a type of hair loss linked to stress, was gentle and effective.

menstrual relief

Some women sail through their periods with nary a mood swing or cramp. Others aren't so lucky. Here are a few comforting yoga poses for that time of the month.

1 If you're experiencing lower back pain, try doing a few knee circles. Lie on your back and bring your knees up toward your chest, keeping your back flat on the floor. Begin to make slow circles with your knees together, gently sweeping them across your abdomen from the right side to the left, continuing around for ten circles.

2 Another good exercise for your back is to kneel, sit back on your heels, and place your arms on the floor close to your body with the palms up. Rest your head on the floor and breathe slowly and deeply, trying to push your exhaled breath into your lower back. Repeat for five breaths, or until the pain subsides.

3 To help ease minor cramps, sit on the floor and bring the soles of your feet together. Grasp them with both hands; be careful not to pull up on your feet. Inhale fully and then lean forward slowly as you exhale, going only as far as feels comfortable while getting a good, gentle stretch in your back and waist. Hold for three to five breaths.

For more relief from cramps, lie on your back and rub your hands together vigorously until they feel warm. Now rest them on your abdomen. Place your right hand below your navel and your left hand above it, and gently rock your torso from side to side for about 20 seconds. Stop rocking and just let your hands rest quietly on your abdomen, visualizing the warmth of your hands soothing any pain. Repeat the exercise a few more times.

To complement these soothing yoga poses, you might want to try some of the aromatherapy measures mentioned at left. Fragrant remedies like these have been used by women for centuries to ease a variety of premenstrual and menstrual woes.

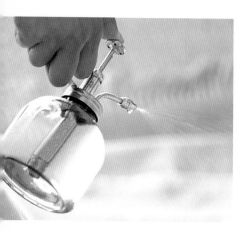

Aromatherapy Menstrual Soothers
To help ease mood swings, scent your room using a spray-mister filled with ten drops of bergamot, lavender, or geranium essential oil and four ounces of water. To help relieve fluid retention, add five drops of patchouli or rosemary essential oil to two teaspoons of carrier oil and massage yourself. To help quiet cramps, add two drops of clary sage or five drops of chamomile essential oil to a bowl of cool water; wet a towel and put it on your abdomen for ten minutes.

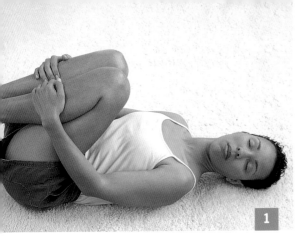

1

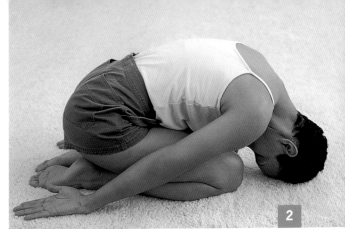

2

3

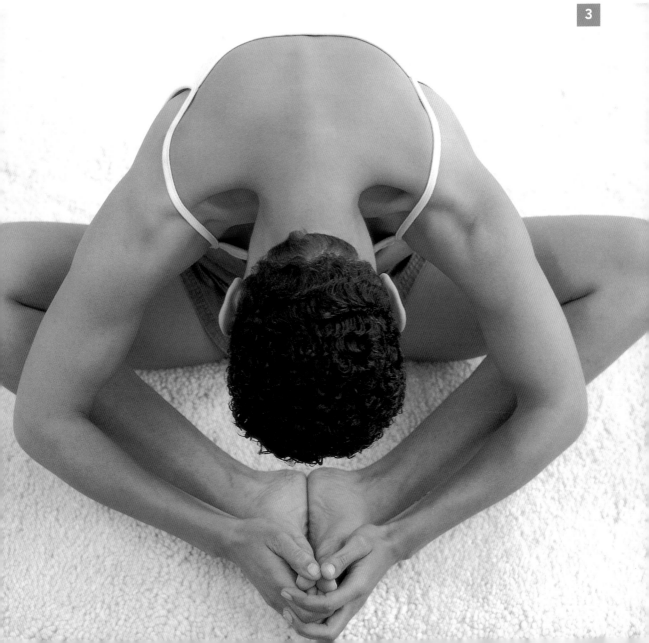

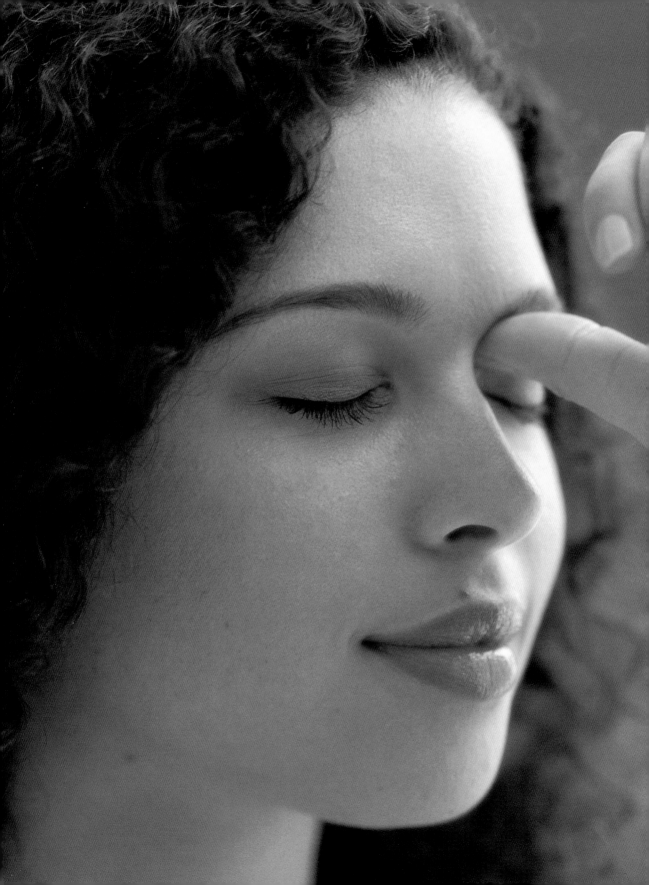

relief for weary eyes

These simple self-massage techniques and focusing
exercises can help dispel headaches, soothe strained
eye muscles, and relax your entire body.

Staring at computer screens, reading small print, and frowning
because you're concentrating (or just plain stressed) can wreak
havoc on your eyes. Some people get headaches, some suffer from
red, irritated eyes, and others find their vision actually starts to blur.
Yoga practitioners, acupuncturists, and massage therapists have long
known that working with the eyes can relieve pent-up tension, both
in the eyes and throughout the rest of the body.

The four exercises described on the following pages are easy to do
and offer quick relief. The trick is having the discipline to stop and
take frequent breaks when you're overworking your eyes—after all,
we develop eyestrain because we're busy, busy, busy! But once you try
these and see what a difference they can make, you're likely to make
the effort. Drawing upon massage, Eastern medicine, and yoga, these
exercises help relax your eye muscles, activate energy meridians (the
channels of energy that healers believe run through the body), and
bring more oxygen to your eyes. Many practitioners maintain that
these methods can improve vision or prevent it from getting worse.

ARE YOU WORKING YOUR EYES TOO HARD?

In order to focus, muscles around the eye have to adjust the shape
of the eye's lens (the part that bends light to create an image on
the retina). To see objects up close, the lens gets thicker. To see
objects far away, the lens gets thinner. People who do a lot of up-
close work (for example, staring at a computer screen or reading
a lot of paperwork) often get eyestrain, which is actually a form of
muscle cramp. Eye exercises relieve the muscles and help them
maintain the ability to change focus easily.

step-by-step sequence ▶

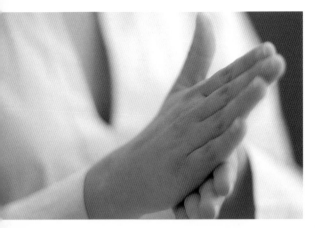

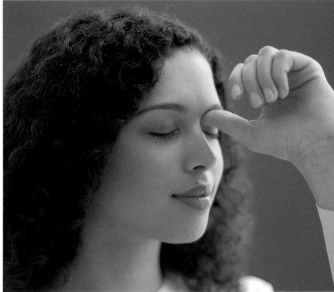

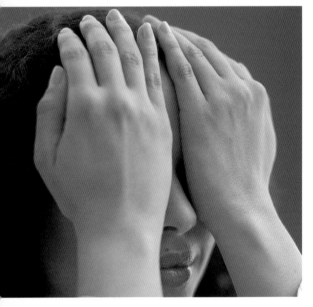

1 To practice eye palming, first wash your hands, then rub them together to warm them. Cup your palms over closed eyes and rest your fingers over your forehead. Apply as much pressure to your eyes as feels comfortable. Breathe deeply. Hold this position for several minutes. (Note: Don't do eye palming if you're wearing contacts.)

2 Close your eyes and press your thumb into the point just beneath your eyebrow and by the bridge of your nose. Press gently upward (be careful: this spot can be sore) for about a minute while breathing deeply. Repeat with the other eye. This sustained pressure helps relieve sore eyes, headaches, blurred vision, and even hay fever.

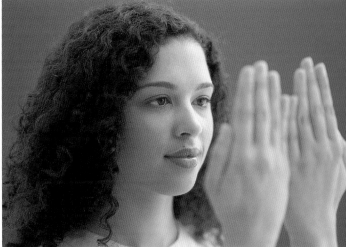

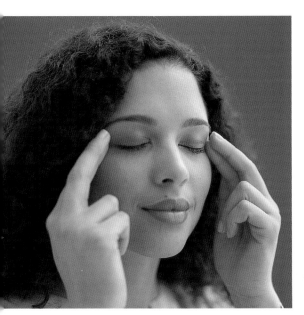

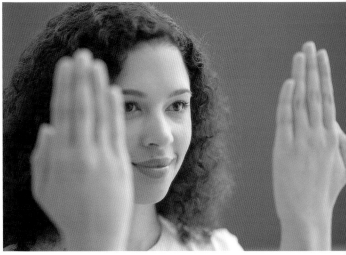

3 Press your fingers into the point at the outside edge of the eye. Lightly massage this area with a circular motion for a few minutes. In both Western and Eastern medical practices, this exercise is believed to improve blood circulation, which can relieve eye tension.

4 To give your eyes a break from constantly focusing on nearby objects, hold your hands about 12 inches in front of your face, with palms in and fingers pointing straight up. As you inhale deeply, move your hands apart and look out at a distant spot. Now exhale and bring your hands together again, readjusting your focus to look at your palms. Alternate between hand positions (and focal points) for two to three minutes.

relieve

head helpers

When stress or fatigue leaves you unable to think straight, these simple moves increase the blood supply to your head, noticeably improving concentration and clarity.

Massage Your Headache Away

Medical practitioners in both Eastern and Western medical traditions recommend massage to relieve headaches—but for very different reasons. Western practitioners believe that when the legions of tiny muscles that hold the skin to the head get too tight, headaches can ensue; therefore a massage can relax those muscles and ease the pain. On the other hand, Eastern practitioners believe that headaches result when energy becomes too congested around the head, disrupting the flow and even distribution of *chi* (energy) that is required for health and wellbeing. They believe a massage can relieve pain because it breaks up this detrimental accumulation.

1 With a rubber-bristled brush, brush your hair back from your hairline with long, firm strokes, moving all the way across your head. Next, hang your head upside down and brush your hair from your neckline to the crown of your head. Repeat both steps five times.

2 Using the pads of your fingertips, scrub slowly and deeply through your hair, all over your scalp. Begin at your forehead and work back over the crown of your head and down to the nape of your neck. After you've massaged your head for a few minutes, you may feel a tingling or pulsing sensation—a sign of increased blood flow, with its burst of brain-stimulating oxygen.

3 Now place your hands on both sides of your head, with the heels of your palms resting on your temples. Gently press your temples for five seconds, then release and glide your hands up to the crown of your head. Repeat the pressing and gliding sequence, varying both the amount of pressure and the speed of your strokes, until you can feel the tension in your head start to ease.

4 Finish your massage by slowly running your fingers through your hair, gently removing any tangles. Then, using light pressure, scratch your scalp with your fingernails, moving from your forehead to the nape of your neck; repeat three times. Each time, increase the pressure slightly. Finally, release any remaining scalp tension by gathering a handful of your hair together and pulling it gently downward. Hold the hair for three seconds before releasing, then move on to another handful of hair. Be sure to gently pull and release all your hair so your entire scalp benefits from the tension relief.

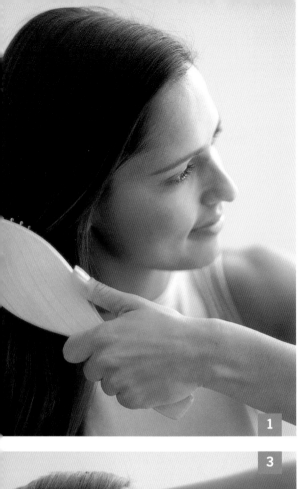

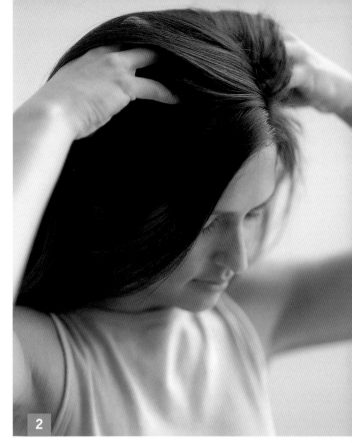

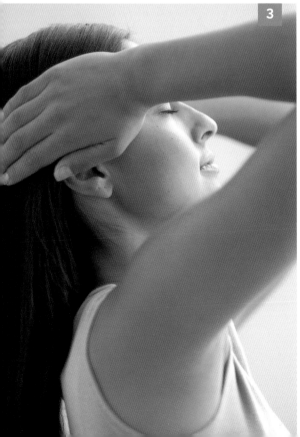

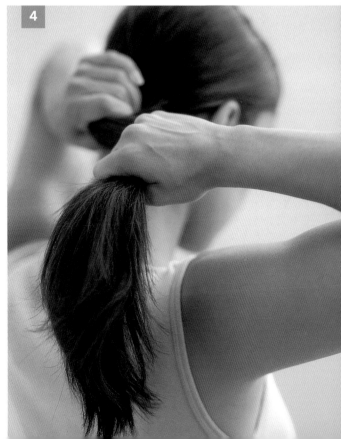

relieve

hearty chicken soup

What Grandma recommends is true: A steaming, fragrant bowl of homemade chicken soup can be just the thing for a head cold, flu, and other maladies.

Ingredients

1 tablespoon extra-virgin olive oil

1 cup chopped onions

1 cup peeled, chopped carrots

½ cup finely chopped celery hearts

1 teaspoon ground cumin

6 cups low-fat, low-sodium chicken broth

1½ cups Yukon gold potatoes, peeled
   and diced into ½-inch pieces

Kosher salt and freshly ground pepper

2 boneless, skinless chicken breast
   halves, cut into ½-inch chunks

2 plum tomatoes, seeded and chopped

8 green beans, cut into ½-inch lengths

½ cup fresh or frozen green peas

2 tablespoons chopped Italian parsley

When you're under the weather, few foods offer as much welcome relief as chicken soup. Not only does the delicious aroma, often evocative of a parent's loving care during childhood, lift our spirits, but the soup itself contains substances that help us feel better. If you like, garnish your steaming bowl of soup with chopped fresh chives.

1 In a large pot over medium-low heat, warm the olive oil and add the onion, carrot, celery, and cumin. Sauté for five to six minutes to soften, but not brown, the vegetables, stirring frequently. Add the chicken broth to the mixture, and bring to a boil.

2 Reduce the heat to very low, and add the potatoes, as well as salt and pepper to taste. Simmer for 15 minutes.

3 Add the chicken chunks, tomatoes, green beans, peas, and parsley. Continue to cook for ten to 15 minutes. Taste the soup and adjust the seasonings. Serve in heated soup bowls.

Serves: 4. Prep time: 20 minutes. Cook time: 35 to 40 minutes.

Nutritional Information Per Serving
Using white chicken meat instead of dark keeps the fat content lower.

Calories	220
Kilojoules	920
Protein	22 g
Carbohydrates	24 g
Total Fat	5 g
Saturated Fat	1 g
Cholesterol	35 mg
Sodium	990 mg
Dietary Fiber	4 g

THE CURE IN THE KITCHEN

Some medical professionals (and lots of grandmas) have been prescribing chicken soup for respiratory ailments for thousands of years. While it might not be an actual *cure* for colds and flus, scientific studies have confirmed that this humble concoction does indeed belong in the medicine cabinet as well as the kitchen, metaphorically speaking. Its anti-inflammatory properties reduce mucus production and help keep airways open. Like other hot liquids, it also breaks up congestion, which helps rid your body more quickly of whatever bacteria or virus is ailing you.

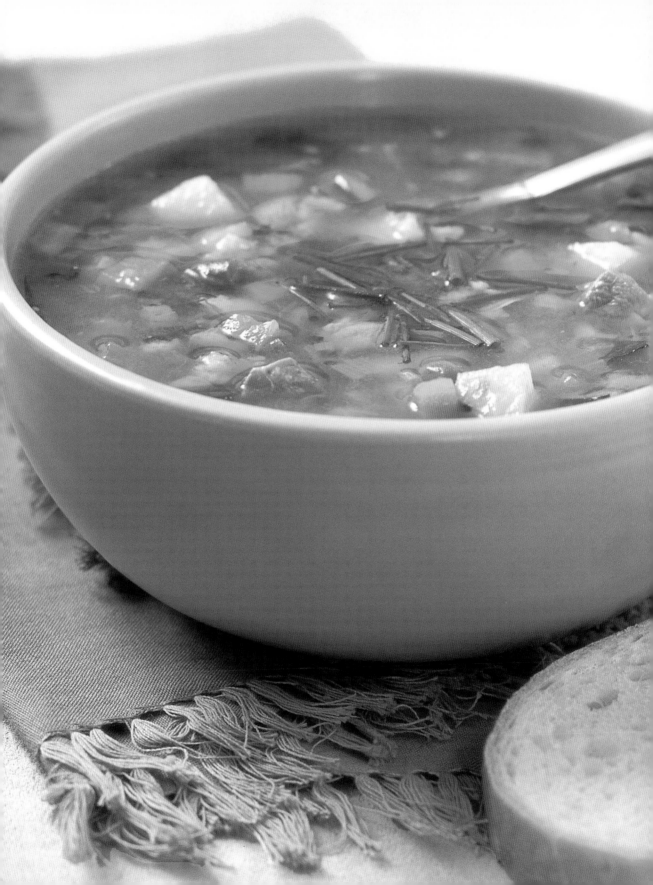

prevent

Like most adages, the saying "An ounce of prevention is worth a pound of cure" contains more than a kernel of truth. But knowing how to prevent various ailments and injuries can be a challenge.

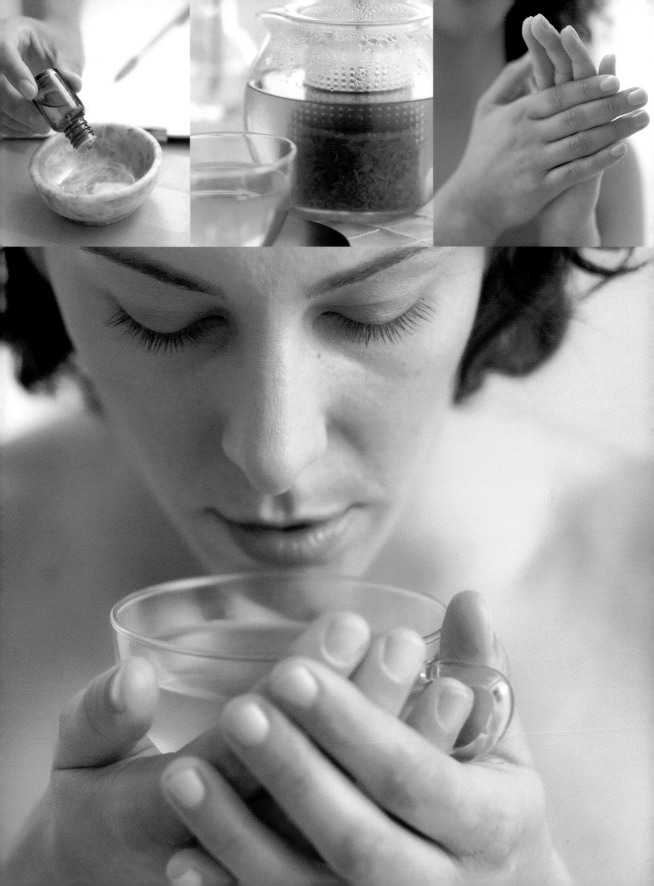

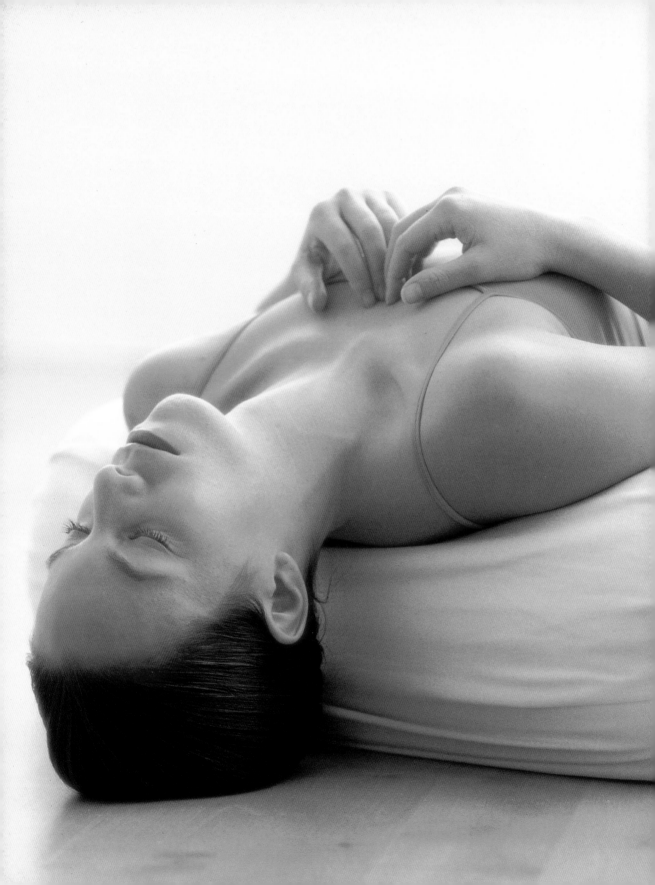

prevent

Some health risks are obvious: We all know that too much sun causes all kinds of damage to our skin, and that too many French fries can do a number on our waistlines and cholesterol levels. Other health risks are more subtle—the fact that sitting on a plane can wreak havoc on your circulatory system, for example, or that a poorly designed computer keyboard can injure your hands.

This chapter will help you deal with some immediate dangers (such as sniffling, sneezing office mates) and help ward off a few potential long-term problems (such as a lack of balance in old age). These measures don't entail anything drastic or complicated; they should fit easily into your lifestyle and appeal to your common sense. You might boost your intake of vitamin C with a fruit smoothie, for instance, to help fortify your immune system. You might massage and stretch your hands and wrists before a long computer session, lessening the risk of developing a repetitive-stress injury. You might enhance your summer glow with a faux tan instead of exposing your skin to the sun's harmful rays. All in all, you might be quite surprised at how easy—and pleasurable—it is to apply that ounce of prevention to help ensure your own wellbeing.

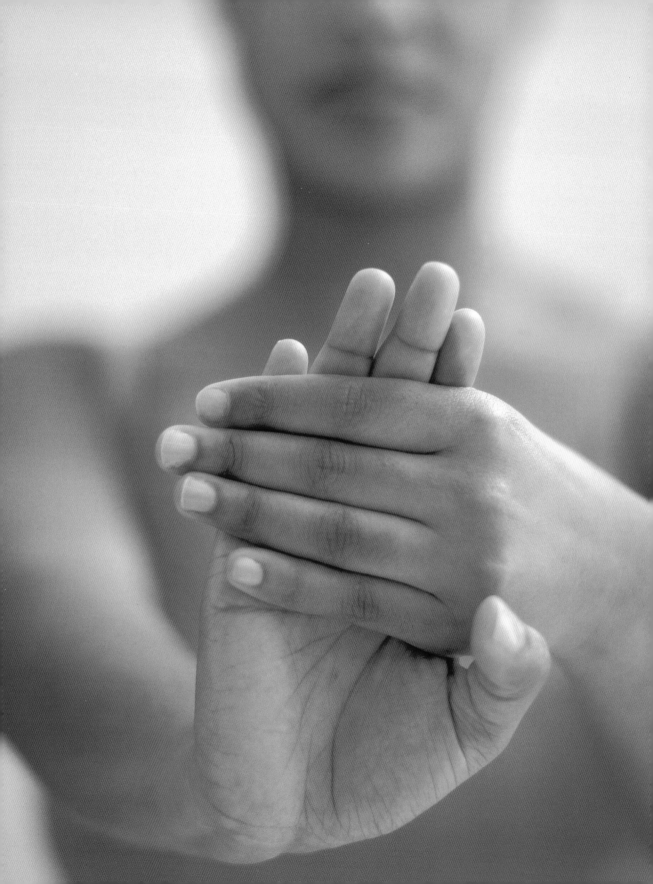

wrist stretches

Protect your hands and wrists with a do-anywhere
exercise to help prevent repetitive-motion problems
and a home remedy to help soothe existing discomfort.

Stretching and massaging your wrist and hand muscles can help make
them more resistant to injury. To begin, sit in a chair and extend your
right arm out in front of you with your palm facing out and your
fingers pointing upward, or rest your right elbow comfortably on a
table, a desktop, or the arm of a chair. Place the fingers of your left
hand horizontally across the fingers of your right hand (see photo at
left) and push the heel of your right hand outward as you gently pull
toward you with your left hand. (Note: If you're not resting your
right elbow on a hard surface, be sure to keep it slightly bent.) Hold
for about ten seconds, then release. Repeat the move on your other
hand. Do only what feels comfortable; you should feel a bit of a
stretch, but be sure to stop at any sign of pain.

If you're already suffering from the effects of a repetitive-stress injury,
such as carpal tunnel syndrome, a witch hazel soak can help relieve
some of the discomfort and stiffness. (Witch hazel has astringent and
anti-inflammatory qualities.) Fill a large bowl with hot water and
add a half cup of witch hazel (see photo at right). Submerge your
hands and wrists in the water for ten minutes. For the first five
minutes, keep your submerged hands still, in any position that feels
comfortable. For the next few minutes, keep your hands submerged
as you alternate between making tight fists and spreading your fingers
wide. Then circle your wrists slowly in both directions, as if you were
holding a pencil and were drawing a spiral in a clockwise direction,
then counterclockwise. In other words, start with small movements
and progress to larger ones; this is more effective at loosening your
wrist muscles than just making the same size circle over and over.
Remove your hands from the water and pat dry.

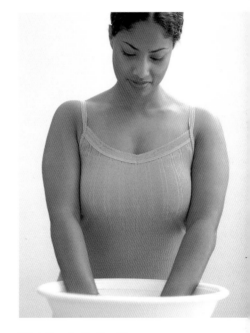

Witch Hazel's Healing Ways
The witch hazel used in this soak has both
astringent and corticoid (anti-inflammatory)
properties. A favorite medicinal plant of
Native Americans, witch hazel has been
used to soothe sore muscles, alleviate the
itch of insect bites, stem bleeding, and
even relieve the pain and swelling of
varicose veins and hemorrhoids.

golden pheasant

This well-known tai chi movement, sometimes called Golden Cock Stands on One Leg, helps you develop balance and stability. It also cultivates an inward focus.

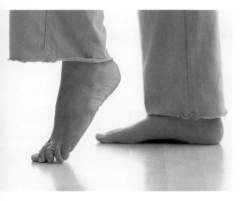

Toe Tips

If you can't keep your balance on one leg (or can't do so without wobbling and hunching your shoulders or tipping forward), rest the toes of one foot gently on the ground. The key is to be relaxed and calm, not stressed by your lack of balance. That will improve with practice.

1 Step out with your right leg and place your right foot at a 45-degree angle. Let your weight settle into your right leg. Keep your spine long and your tailbone tucked in.

2 Bending your knee, slowly lift your left leg as high as you can while still keeping a soft angle to your knee, and point your toes down. Raise your left arm, bending the elbow up softly. Point your fingers straight up with the palm facing inward. Keep your right arm down and slightly bent by your side, with your palm facing the ground. Focus on a fixed point in the distance to help maintain your balance. Keep your shoulders relaxed and down, soften all your body angles, and maintain a straight line from the crown of your head to the bottom of your torso. As you do this exercise, think of a bird showing off his plumage and try to keep yourself as upright and elegant as possible. Do the sequence on the other side. Then repeat the Golden Pheasant on both sides once more.

STRIKE A BALANCE

Tai chi's fluid, weight-shifting movements help strengthen leg muscles, maintain bone density, enhance joint flexibility, and promote a good sense of balance and body awareness. All of these benefits can mean fewer falls, an especially important consideration as we age; a recent survey conducted by Rhode Island hospitals estimated that one out of three seniors takes a tumble at least once a year. Just how effective is tai chi at preventing falls? Researchers at Emory University in Georgia found that senior citizens who take tai chi lessons once a week and practice for 15 minutes twice daily can cut their risk of falls nearly in *half*.

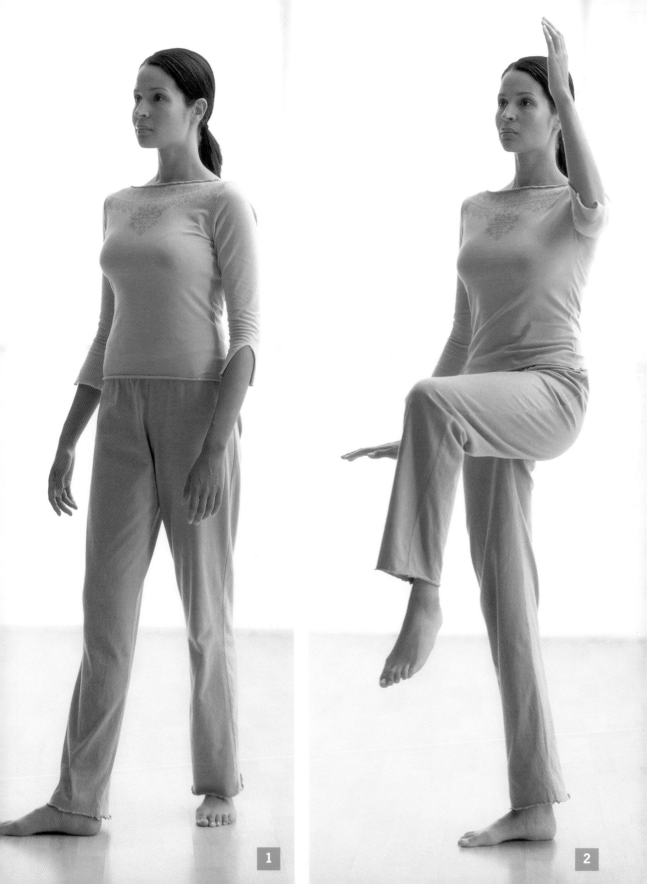

posture awareness

Pilates helps you develop good posture, which is the gateway to a range of benefits—from making you feel more graceful to preventing back injury.

"Stand Up Straight!"

That's an admonition that most of us heard countless times as we were growing up, and it turns out to be excellent advice. Correct posture is important to both our health and our appearance. It opens up our chest, allowing our lungs to take deep, long breaths; it keeps our spine straight, relieving pressure on the vertebrae; and it helps prevent back problems later in life. A beauty bonus: Good posture can also make us look much more graceful and elegant.

How do you know when you are maintaining proper posture? This Pilates-inspired exercise can help. Use it as a meditation on alignment, as well as a way to correct your posture throughout the day.

1 Stand with your feet hip-width apart, arms relaxed by your sides, and toes pointing straight ahead. Check what Pilates teachers call the "triad of the foot"—the even distribution of weight among the ball of your big toe, the ball of your little toe, and the back edge of your heel. Focus on the lines from your inner ankle bones, up the inside of your legs, to the pubic bone; imagine a slight magnetic force attracting these lines together. Lift the muscles of your pelvic floor, as if you were controlling urination. Draw your belly button in toward the spine. Position your ribs on top of your pelvis and lengthen your spine. Drop your shoulders down and back, and then widen your collarbones. Tuck in your chin slightly. Take a long breath; notice how your body feels when everything is aligned properly.

2 Keeping your weight balanced on the triad of the foot, drop your head and let your body roll down vertebra by vertebra, as far as you are comfortable, softly bending your knees. Dangle your hands in front of you. Pause for a moment, and then bring yourself back up slowly, lengthening as you rise. Feel the segments of your body stack up on top of each other, one after the other.

3 Now float your arms over your head. Lengthen your spine and arch backward (as far as is comfortable), again being conscious of keeping your weight on the triad of the foot. Pause, then return to an upright position, feeling your body align itself with your ribs on top of your pelvis and with the abdominals tight; slowly bring your arms down along your sides. Repeat the exercise two more times.

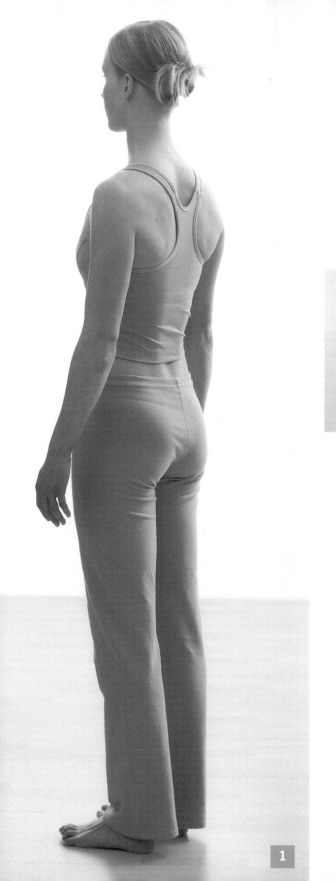

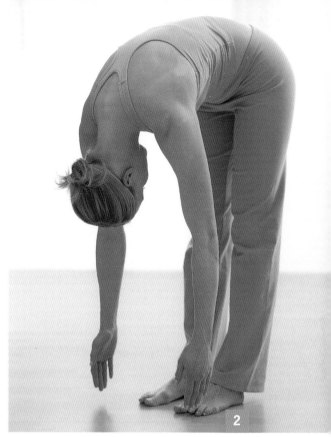

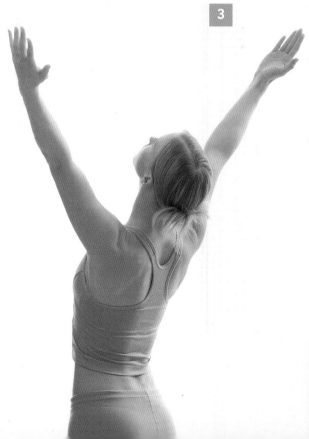

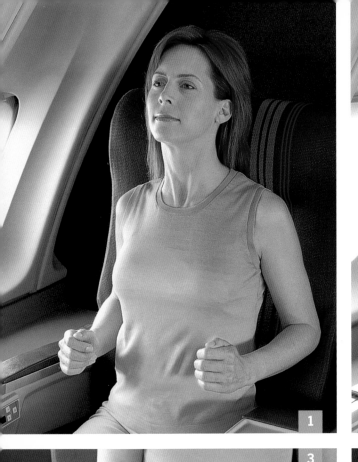

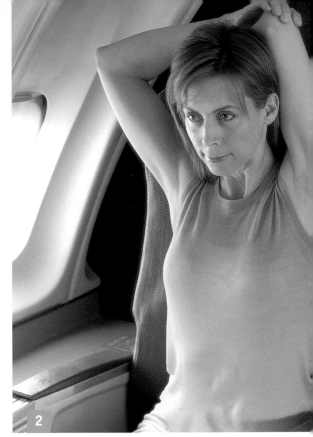

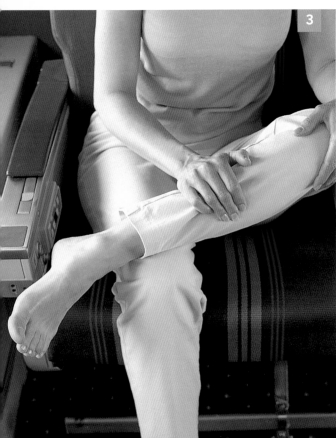

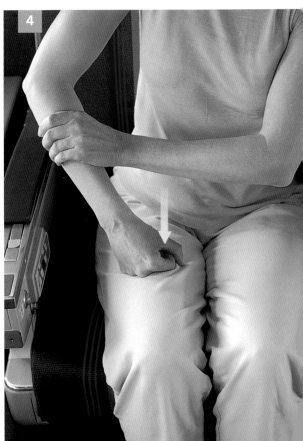

in-flight workout

Sitting for long periods can cause muscles to stiffen and impede blood circulation. Head off problems with stretches you can do discreetly in your airplane seat.

1 To encourage deeper breathing and perk up sluggish circulation, press both elbows firmly back into your seat, arch your chest forward, and inhale and exhale three times while maintaining the pressure with your arms. Relax, rounding your back slightly. Repeat three to five times, until you feel your heart pumping a little.

2 Now raise both arms over your head, bend your elbows, and grasp your left elbow with your right hand. Take a deep breath, then exhale and gently pull your left elbow to the right. Lean a little to the right and try to extend the stretch down to your waist. Hold for about two seconds, then sit up straight, rest your arms on top of your head as you inhale deeply, and repeat the stretch as you exhale, going a few inches farther each time. Then stretch your right side.

3 Improve the circulation in your legs by using the sports massage technique of compression (see page 129 ◄). Rest one ankle on top of the opposite thigh. Firmly press the heel of your hand into your calf with rhythmic, pumping strokes, working the muscles from ankle to knee. Then increase the blood flow to your legs by pointing your toes down and then up. Flex each foot this way about a dozen times.

4 Hold your right forearm with your left hand. Position the top of your right fist just above your right knee. Now press down on your right leg with the flat of your knuckles, bending your body forward for added strength. Release, move your fist an inch or so toward your hip, and repeat. Cover your entire thigh this way, rhythmically rocking your weight forward and back. Then switch sides and repeat on your other leg. During long flights (or car or bus rides), try to perform all of these steps every two hours or so.

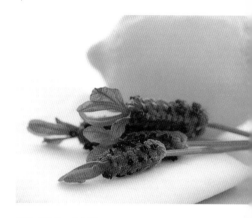

Help for Fearful Fliers

If the thought of getting on a plane makes your heart race, try this technique to take the edge off your fears: Put a couple of cotton pads sprinkled with a few drops of lavender and lemon essential oils in a small resealable plastic bag, and carry it on board with you. If you start to feel anxious, open the bag and inhale the comforting scent released by the aromatic oils. Close your eyes, concentrate on breathing slowly and deeply, and meditate for a few minutes.

immunity boost

By stimulating the lymphatic and endocrine systems and quieting the central nervous system, regular yoga practice can help keep you healthy and fit.

Yoga and the Immune System
A number of international studies have shown that several stress hormones, including adrenaline, cortisol, and noradrenaline, have a negative impact on the immune system and impair the function of T cells, white blood cells, and aptly named natural killer cells, all of which help the body prevent and fight infection. Yoga, because of its meditative, calming nature, induces relaxation, consequently stemming the release of stress hormones. It also encourages the production of endorphins, which boost the immune system, reduce pain, and activate the brain's so-called pleasure centers.

1 Stand with your feet together and your arms hanging loosely by your sides. Begin to twist your torso gently from side to side, allowing your arms to swing and bump lightly against your body. Gradually increase your speed so that the force of your swings lifts your arms away from your body. Continue for a minute or two to stimulate the lymph glands in your underarms. Then stand and rest in the Mountain pose (see page 248 ►).

2 Now lie on your back next to an unobstructed wall. Your back should be perpendicular to the wall, and your knees should be slightly bent. Keeping your buttocks pressed against the wall, swing both legs up against the wall, settle your back on the floor, and rest your arms on the floor with your palms up. Align your body so your shoulders square up with your hips; your arms will angle out from your body alongside your hips. Hold for one to five minutes, as comfort allows. To come out of the pose, let your knees sink slowly toward your chest, and roll to one side.

3 Place a bolster, firm pillow, or rolled-up blanket on the floor and lie down so that it supports your upper back while the top of your head dangles back and touches the floor. (Make sure this angle is not too severe, especially if you have neck or back problems; you don't want to put any undue strain on your neck.) Keep your legs together, and gently drum your fingertips on your breastbone (the center of your chest) to stimulate your thymus gland, an important regulator in the body's immune system. Hold for about one minute, then use your arms to raise yourself into a sitting position.

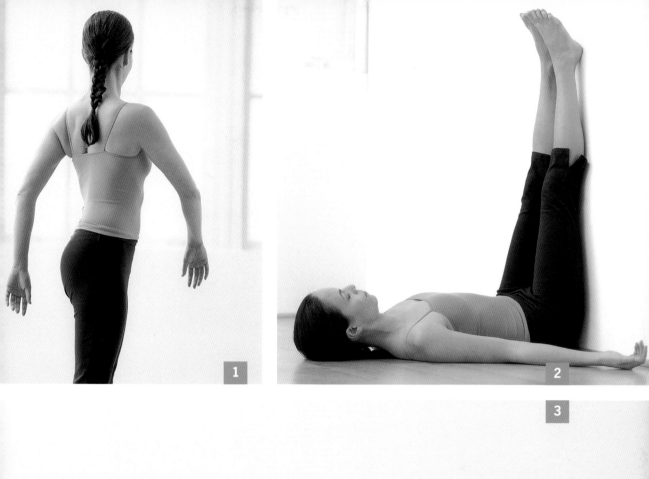

1

2

3

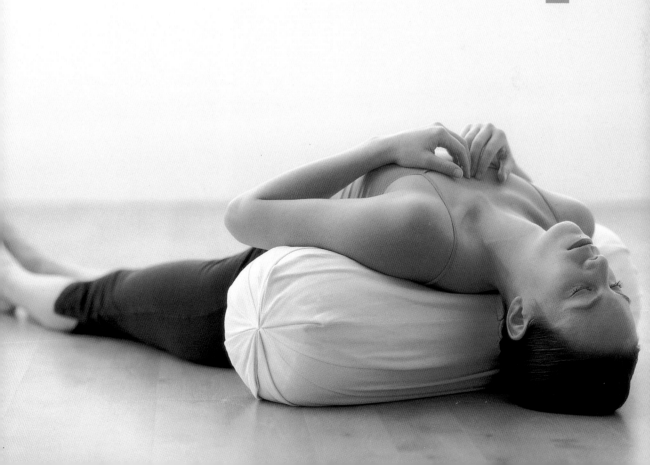

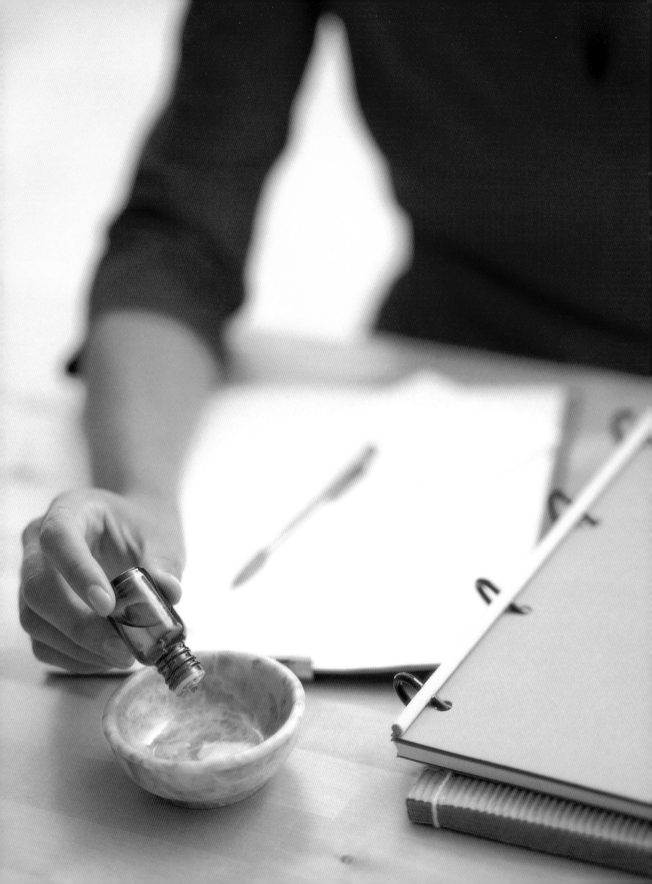

office aromatherapy

Keep office germs at bay with a variety of potent and aromatic essential oils that have long-proven antibacterial and antiviral properties.

Most workplaces are, by their very nature, bad for our health. All those colleagues, customers, and clients sneezing and coughing, all that stale air circulating and recirculating—no wonder workers come down with illness after illness. In fact, one internationally known researcher in design and environmental analysis found that people who worked in offices with modern air-conditioning and heating systems had twice as many upper-respiratory illnesses as those who worked in buildings with natural ventilation.

You may not be able to fling open your windows or persuade your coworkers to stay home when they're under the weather, but you can enlist a powerful ally in the fight against office germs: essential oils. A good number of them have been shown to possess antibacterial, antifungal, and antiviral properties. The aromas of most of these oils also have beneficial psychological effects and, in some cases, are reputed to help boost the immune system.

Germ-killing essential oils include thyme, tea tree, spike lavender, pine, fir, rosemary, and eucalyptus. Diffusing these scents throughout your office is an excellent way to activate their therapeutic qualities. Electric diffusers (see page 139 ◄) are best for this purpose because there's little risk of overheating the oils, thus destroying some of their potency, and they circulate the scent efficiently. You also can add a few drops of your chosen essential oil to a little water in a small bowl and place it in your work space, or drizzle a few drops onto cotton balls and put them near (but not on) a radiator or heating vent. One good-neighbor caveat: Keep in mind that the fragrance you find delightful might seem downright offensive to your office mates. Ask your coworkers if they mind any of the oils you use, and try to pick a few that everyone finds appealing (or at least inoffensive).

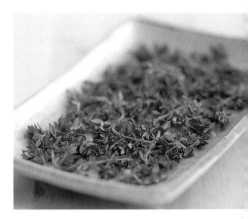

A Quadruple Threat
With its antiseptic, antibacterial, antiviral, and antifungal properties, thyme (pictured above) is one of the most potent germ-killers in the aromatherapist's arsenal. Be careful, though: While appropriate for use in a diffuser, the type of thyme essential oil containing carvacrol (a powerful antiseptic) is too harsh to be directly applied to skin.

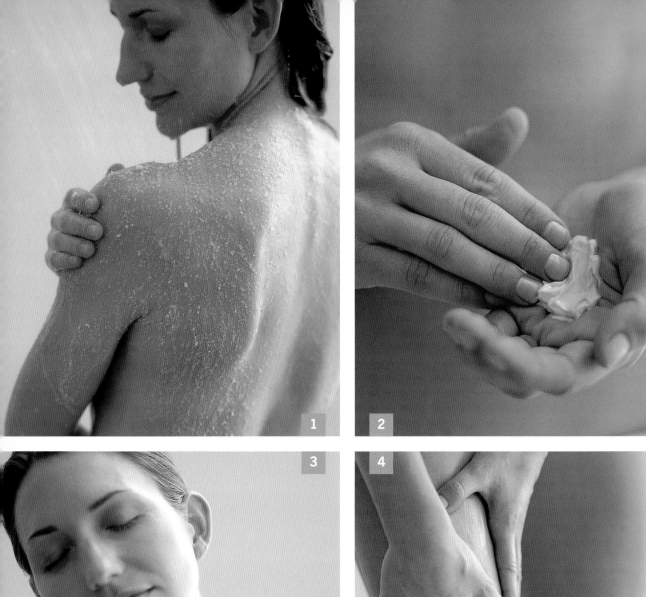
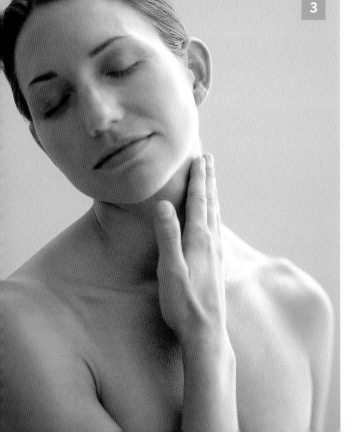
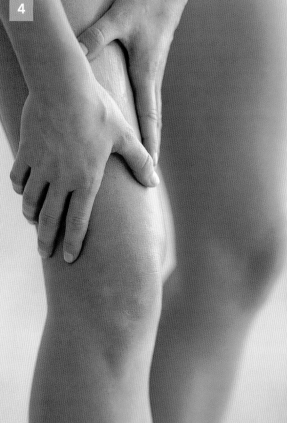

self-tanning

You love the look of tanned skin but know better than
to bake in the sun. Avoid the burn and get your glow by
using lotions that activate your skin's natural pigment.

1 Prepare your skin by using an exfoliating scrub (see page 59 ◄)
to remove dead skin cells; this will help prevent streaking or uneven
color. Shower off afterward and dry your body completely.

2 Squeeze a dollop of self-tanning lotion into the palm of one hand
(consider wearing disposable gloves). Rub your hands together lightly,
just enough to cover your palms and fingertips with the product.
Don't be fooled by the light color; the lotion works not by dyeing
your skin bronze but by triggering the melanin-producing cells that
give your skin its natural golden glow when exposed to the sun.

3 For an all-over tan, begin applying the self-tanner evenly and
sparingly to your face, neck, shoulders, and chest. Use smooth,
circular strokes and massage in well to avoid blotching and streaking.
It's better to apply a few thin coats than to plaster on the product.
Be careful not to get any lotion in your eyes.

4 Move on to your arms, backs of your hands, torso, back (you
might need a friend to help you with your back), legs, and tops of
your feet. Remember to rub in the self-tanner thoroughly and apply
it as evenly as you can. Watch out for easy-to-miss spots, such as the
back of your knees and hands, or for any extra lotion that might
settle in between your toes or in bony areas such as your ankles and
shins. If you're wearing gloves, remove them and apply the lotion
evenly to your hands. Otherwise, wash your hands immediately. Let
the lotion dry for about 30 minutes before dressing to avoid staining
your clothing. You can reapply the lotion daily until you obtain the
shade you desire. The color will fade as your skin cells exfoliate.

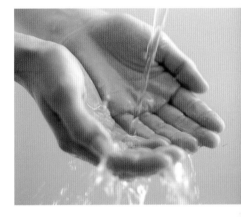

All Washed Up
We can't stress this enough: Be sure to
wash your hands thoroughly with soap
and water immediately after applying
self-tanning lotion. If you don't, your
hands will absorb too much of the lotion
and you'll end up with dark, streaked
palms—probably not the effect you
were after. Another option is to wear
disposable gloves, which come with
some kits, while applying the lotion.

tea time

A simple cup of tea has long been used to warm the body and soothe the nerves. Today researchers believe the brew also helps prevent a variety of illnesses.

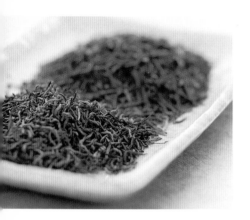

Loose or Bags?
The health benefits are the same whether you use loose tea or tea bags. Steep your tea for at least three minutes to release the antioxidants and other helpful substances.

Introduced in China some 4,000 years ago, tea is the most popular beverage in the world after water, and one that many people favor instinctively when they're ill or feeling frazzled. This is a good thing: Scientists now know that tea offers a cupful of health benefits.

The leaves of black, green, white, and oolong teas (that is, any tea derived from the evergreen *Camellia sinensis,* which doesn't include herbal varieties) are rich in chemicals called polyphenols, which contain the antioxidants that may combat illnesses including heart disease and several types of cancer. Recent research at Harvard Medical School shows that the amino acid L-theanine, which is found in tea, boosts the body's defenses against bacterial, viral, fungal, and parasitic infections. Other research has found that tea can protect against osteoporosis and some kinds of allergies. Iced and hot tea have equal amounts of antioxidants, but beware of some bottled teas, as their antioxidant levels can be low and their sugar content high.

THE TYPES OF TEA

The media's trumpeting of tea's many health benefits has resulted in an explosion of exotic varieties available in stores and online. But consumers sometimes are confused about the many differences among the main varieties. Here's a quick guide to help you sort out your tea options.

TYPE	PROCESSING TECHNIQUE	CHARACTERISTICS
Black (also known as red tea)	Still-green leaves are withered, then rolled. Oxidation darkens leaves. Dried in ovens.	Flavors from nutty and spicy to flowery. Accounts for about 90 percent of tea consumption in the Western world.
Green	Leaves are allowed to wither, then are steamed or pan-fried, rolled, and dried. No oxidation.	Light, slightly bitter, grassy flavors. Most popular tea in Asia.
White	Leaves with white down are picked, steamed, and dried. No oxidation. Dried by pan-frying.	Delicate, complex, and sweet flavors. The rarest and most expensive tea.
Oolong	After withering, leaves are bruised and allowed to partially oxidize. Dried by pan-frying.	Fragrant and naturally sweet flavors. Properties are somewhere between the black and green teas.

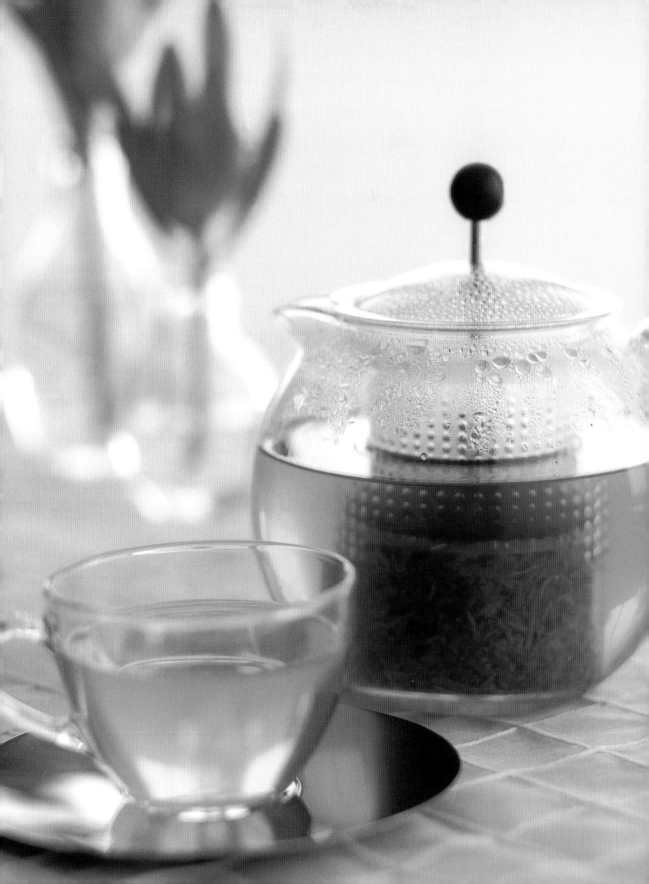

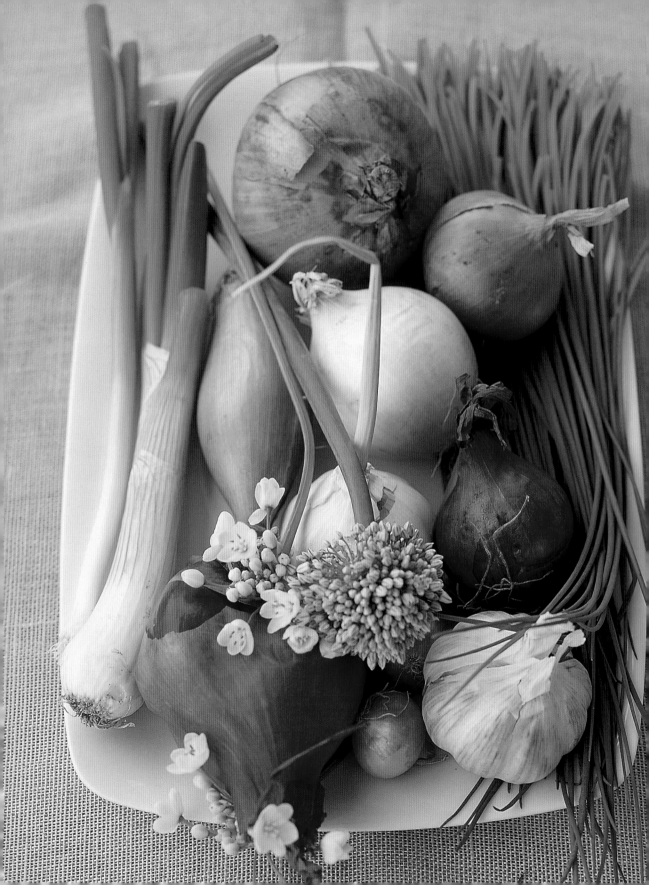

phytochemicals

Upping your daily intake of fruits and vegetables can help your body fight off diseases, thanks to some special substances found in plants ranging from onions to berries.

Most dietary guidelines recommend that plant-based foods—such as fresh fruits, vegetables, and grains—should make up the bulk of what you consume. That's partly because they're high in fiber and nutrients, but it's also because they contain hordes of substances causing a lot of buzz in the scientific community: phytochemicals.

Phytochemicals (the first two syllables are pronounced FIGHT-oh) are naturally occurring plant chemicals that seem to fight or protect against many major types of disease, including diabetes, cancer, heart disease, hypertension, osteoporosis, arthritis, urinary-tract infections, and vision problems. These substances are believed to ward off cell damage, stimulate the immune system, aid the body's detoxification mechanisms, and perhaps even slow down the aging process. Since 1980, phytochemicals have been the subject of many studies focusing on precisely how they work and how else they may benefit our health. One thing scientists already are sure about: Phytochemicals work in conjunction with each other, as well as nutrients and dietary fiber, in complex, overlapping ways. That makes it difficult—perhaps even impossible—to reproduce their effects with supplements, so you can't just pop a pill, you have to eat the foods.

To date, researchers have identified more than 900 types of these valuable chemicals in food, and estimate that you may consume more than 100 kinds of phytochemicals in a single serving of vegetables. Dietary guidelines vary widely, but most health authorities seem to recommend eating five to ten servings of fruits and vegetables a day. This sounds like a lot, but there are many sources of phytochemicals from which to choose. Just think about eating a rainbow of foods; bright colors usually signal the presence of phytochemicals.

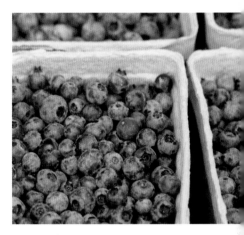

A Rainbow of Wonders
Blueberries are rich in phenols, terpenes, and ellagic acid, phytochemicals that are thought to enhance the immune system, help prevent cancer, and decrease blood cholesterol levels. Other dark red, blue, and purple vegetables and fruits, such as plums, beets, and purple grapes, also contain these disease-fighting compounds.

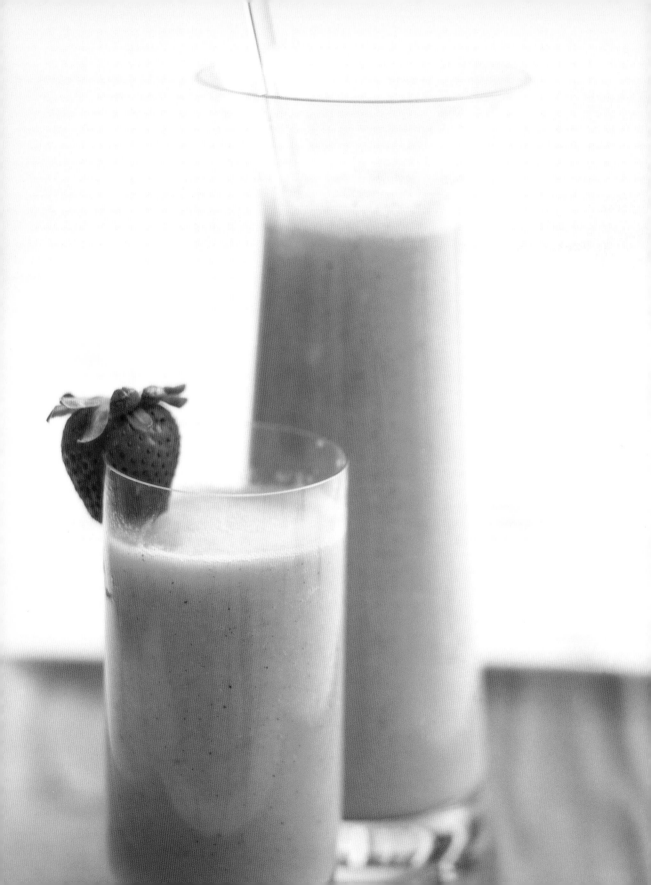

vitamin c smoothie

A fruit-packed smoothie rich in this crucial vitamin provides plenty of power to your immune system, as well as a tantalizing tang for your taste buds.

Starting in the late 1970s, Dr. Linus Pauling advocated taking megadoses of vitamin C to ward off colds. That's not considered scientifically valid anymore, but researchers do believe the vitamin stimulates the production and activity of various components of the immune system, which means it might help prevent a wide range of ailments, including diabetes, infections, and osteoporosis. As an antioxidant, vitamin C also slows the damage from free radicals—unstable and reactive substances found in the body that have been linked to heart disease, cancer, and other illnesses.

How much vitamin C should you take? The U.S. Food and Drug Administration recommends 75 to 125 milligrams per day. You can get that from a range of foods, including fruits such as citrus, berries, and melons, and vegetables such as cabbage and other greens.

Drinking a fresh fruit smoothie is an easy way to boost your vitamin C intake. Combine the ingredients listed at right in a blender and blend at high speed until smooth. If you're using fresh fruit, add ice.

Ingredients

¾ cup orange juice

½ cup fresh or frozen mango chunks

½ cup fresh or frozen strawberries

½ cup chopped kiwi

½ cup low-fat vanilla yogurt

½ cup ice (optional)

- Serves: 1
- Prep time: 5 minutes

Nutritional Information Per Serving

Oranges and mangoes contain folic acid, an immune-system booster.

Calories	310
Kilojoules	1,290
Protein	9 g
Carbohydrates	67 g
Total Fat	2.5 g
Saturated Fat	1 g
Cholesterol	5 mg
Sodium	80 mg
Dietary Fiber	6 g

BEAUTY BONUSES

Vitamin C is renowned for being a powerful antioxidant that helps protect skin from free radicals, which form in the presence of environmental pollution and sunlight. These free radicals, in turn, break down the skin's collagen and elastin, both of which help keep the skin firm. When used in cleansers and moisturizers, vitamin C is credited with strengthening those deep layers of skin, which can reduce the appearance of wrinkles and make skin firmer. One tip: Vitamin C loses its potency quickly, so look for products sold in dark glass bottles or metal tubes, which protect the vitamin from light.

retreat

We all need to seek sanctuary from time to time, to step back and replenish our physical and emotional strength. Indeed, sometimes making a tactical retreat can be the best way to move forward.

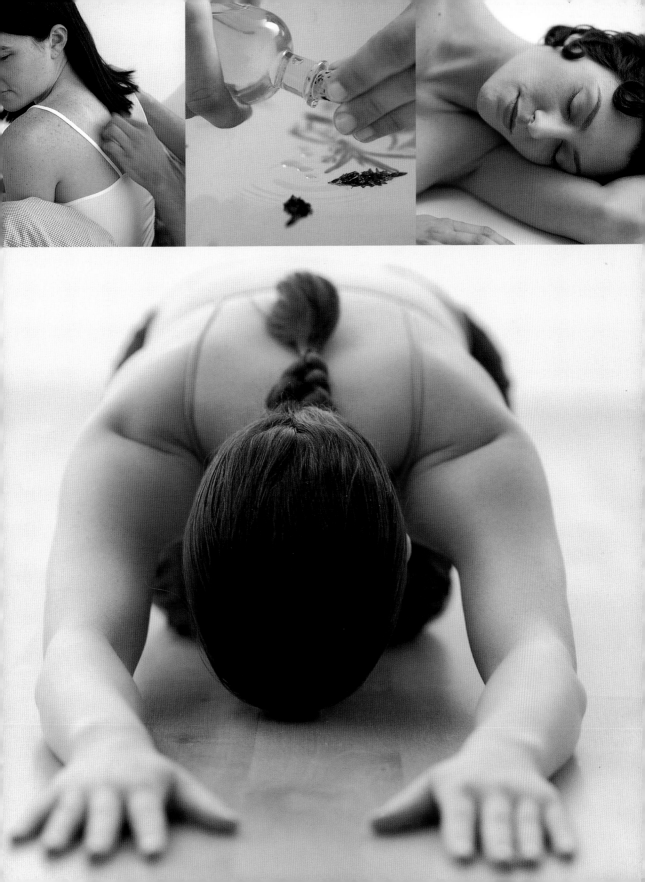

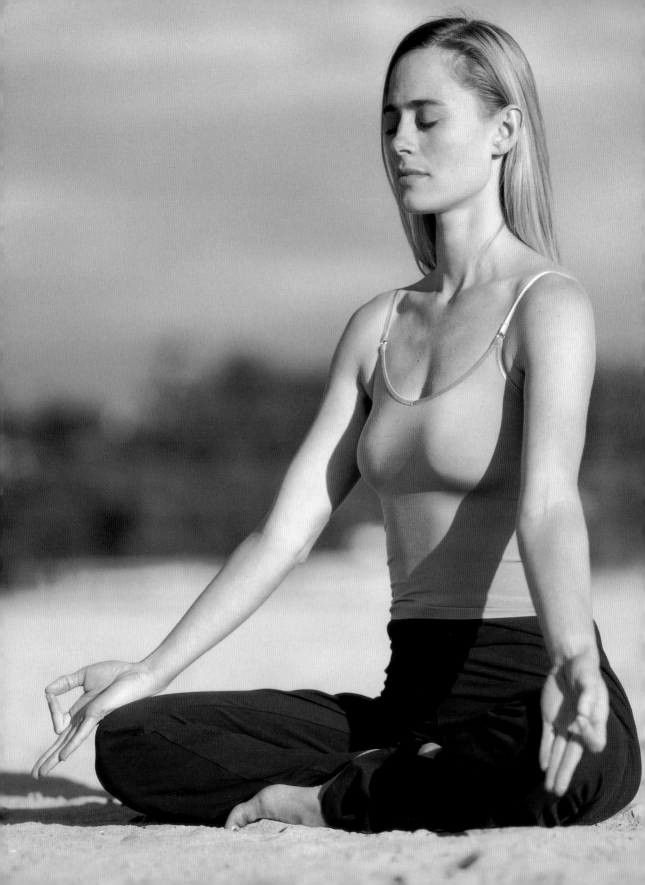

retreat

All women need to stage occasional escapes from the barrages of
sensory stimulation, professional duties, and social obligations that
fill our worlds. We need to unwind, we need to regroup, we just
need to rest. Once the mind is still and the heart is calm, insights
emerge and decisions work themselves out more easily.

Some of us simply close the bathroom door and soak in an
aromatic warm bath. Others walk along a deserted shoreline or
meditate in a secluded garden. Another approach is to take a more
formal refuge, perhaps in a yoga center or other haven devoted to
relaxation. Whichever path you choose, a retreat lets you escape
the chaos of the outside world and focus on the universe within,
reconnecting with your physical, emotional, and spiritual selves.

Use the ideas on the following pages to defuse stress and promote
self-awareness. You also might experiment with retreats of your own
making, whether they involve reading a book in a grassy meadow,
attending a prayer service, or heading off on a solo weekend at an
isolated inn. The point is to relax, release, and reflect, so you can
move ahead with clarity and a sense of wellbeing.

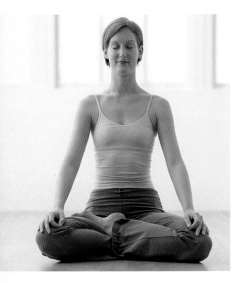

alternate nostril breath

This ancient yoga practice is said to calm and balance physical and mental energies, making it especially helpful for relaxing before meditation or sleep.

Sit in a comfortable position, either in a chair or on the floor. Keep your back straight and your chin up. Begin to breathe deeply and regularly, and try to empty your mind of conscious thoughts.

When you're ready to begin alternate nostril breathing, fold the index and middle fingers of your right hand into your right palm. Close your right nostril with your thumb and exhale through your left nostril. Now inhale slowly and fully through your left nostril.

Now, using the same hand, close your left nostril with your ring and little fingers. Release your thumb and exhale through your right nostril. Then inhale through your right nostril and switch again.

Continue this pattern (exhaling and inhaling through one side and then switching to the other) for one to five minutes.

Half-Lotus Pose

When sitting and meditating, beginners often just sit cross-legged. When you get more proficient, you might want to try the Half-Lotus pose pictured above. Sitting up tall, gently lift one foot and place it on the opposite thigh, sole up and close to your hip. Tuck the other foot under its opposite thigh. One leg might be more comfortable in the upper position than the other.

TWO SIDES TO THE STORY

Brain researchers have confirmed what yogis have long espoused: that when you're breathing through your right nostril, the electrical activity in the brain's left hemisphere is stimulated, and when you breathe through your left nostril, the right hemisphere is fired up.

LEFT HEMISPHERE CONTROLS:	RIGHT HEMISPHERE CONTROLS:
• Analytical reasoning	• Intuitive thought
• Language	• Creativity
• Mathematical ability	• Aesthetic sensibilities
• Application of order and patterns	• Perception of order and patterns
• Focusing on details	• Focusing on the big picture

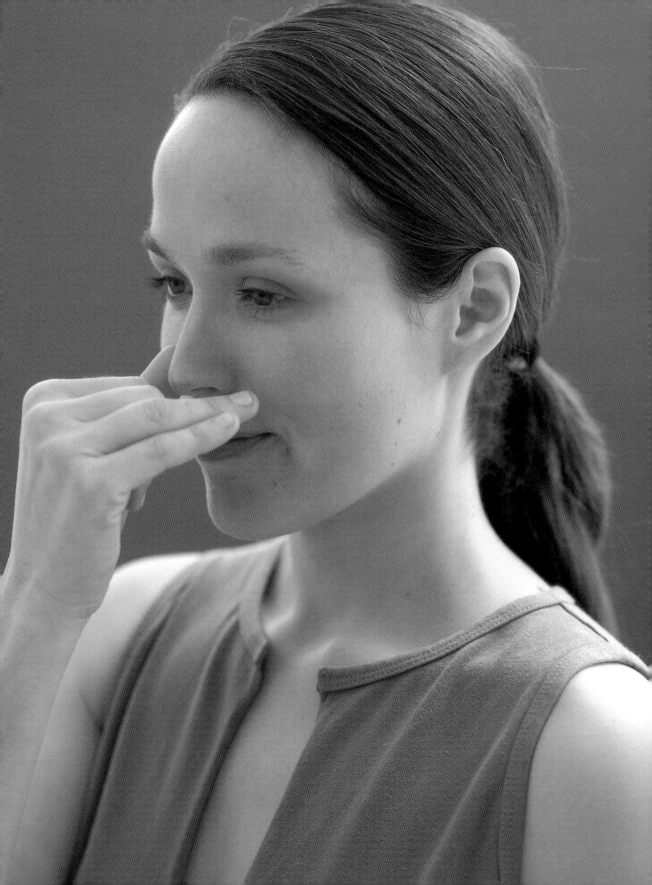

diamonds

Unwinding before bedtime often results in a better night's sleep. Try these Diamond yoga poses to calm your mind and release tension built up during the day.

Less Rest for the Weary
In the United States, the average time spent sleeping on weeknights is now about seven hours, compared with the nine hours folks were getting in the early 20th century. That change is resulting in serious consequences. Inadequate sleep has been linked to diabetes, hypertension, and hormonal disruption, as well as anger, stress, and sadness. So how much sleep is enough? Many experts say eight hours per night for most people.

1 To perform the Upward Triple Diamond pose, lie on your back in bed, bring the soles of your feet together, and let your knees sink down. Raising your arms overhead with your palms facing up, bring your thumbs and index fingers together. Let the weight of your arms and legs sink downward, bringing a sense of release to your hips and shoulders. As your body relaxes, feel your mind begin to empty. Hold for one minute, paying careful attention to your breathing and keeping worries and other disturbing thoughts at bay, then release.

2 To further your retreat from the world, lie facedown and lift your arms overhead in preparation for the Downward Triple Diamond. Bring your thumbs and index fingers together, palms down. Bend your knees, then slide them apart and bring the soles of your feet together. Relax your hips; for greater intensity, you can gently press your feet downward. Hold for ten breaths, drawing your mind deeply inward. Lift your feet and bring your legs together to release.

A BEDTIME STORY

If you often have trouble going to sleep (or staying asleep), a few lifestyle changes may help make your body and mind more receptive to a good night's rest. Perhaps the most important thing you can do is to establish a relaxing bedtime routine, such as drinking a cup of chamomile tea, listening to soothing music, reading, or meditating. Here are some other ideas for getting a little more shut-eye each evening.

TOP TIPS FOR BETTER SLEEP

- Establish a regular schedule for going to sleep and waking up.
- Don't eat heavy or spicy meals within three hours of bedtime.
- Drink alcohol in moderation, and never within two hours of going to bed.
- Promise yourself that you'll deal with worries tomorrow—just not right now.
- Make your bedroom a haven for sleep; don't do work or watch TV in bed.
- Avoid vigorous exercise within five hours of sleeping.
- Empty your bladder before crawling into bed.
- Avoid caffeine in the afternoon or evening hours.
- If you wake up and can't get back to sleep, read until you feel drowsy.

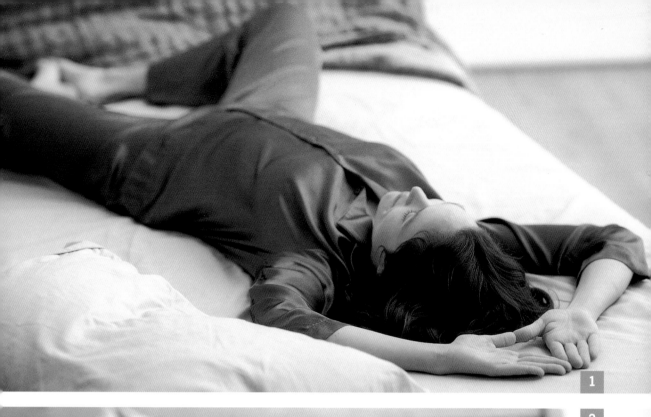

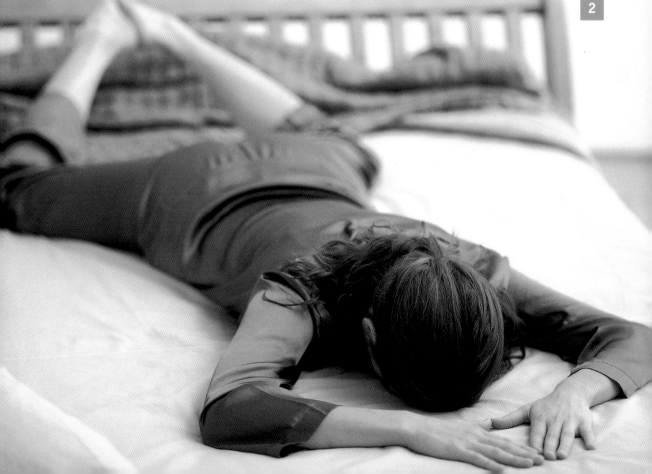

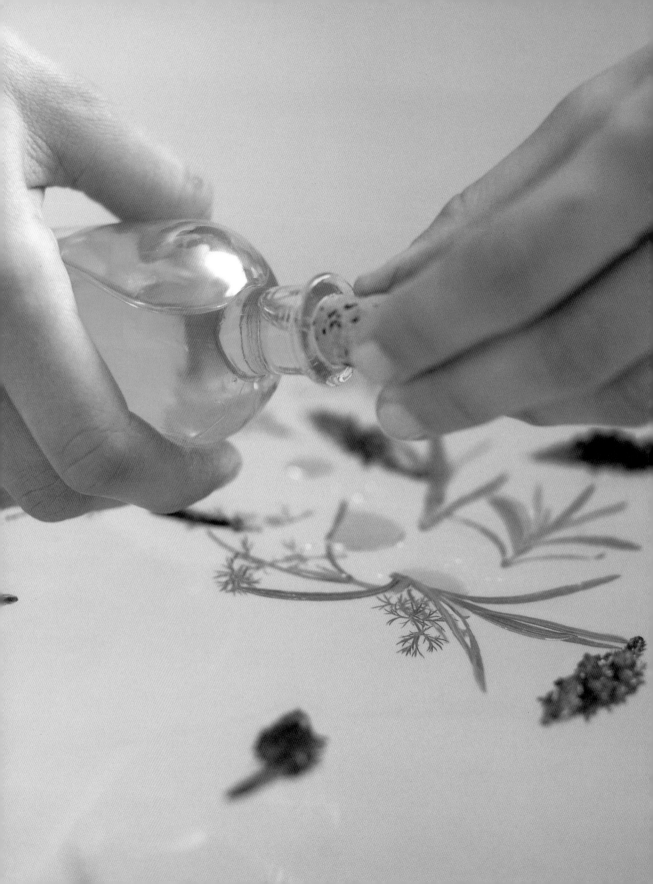

lavender bath

Evocative of the fields of Provence, lavender is the most popular essential oil. A bath scented with this calming fragrance is sure to soothe both the skin and the spirit.

To dissolve away the cares of the day, run a warm bath. Don't make the water too hot or you'll just end up feeling drained, not relaxed. Add five to seven drops of lavender essential oil blended with one ounce of carrier oil, or create a blend of lavender and other soothing essential oils (see recipe at right). After the bath has been filled, stir the water with your hand to evenly distribute the oil; you don't want it to pool on top, as it might cause skin irritation. Light one or several scented candles and set them around the bathroom, and then dim or turn off the bathroom lights. Lie back in the warm water, preferably using a bath pillow so you can truly unwind.

Close your eyes and let your mind empty of the chatter of the day. Take a mental inventory of your body, starting with the top of your head and slowly moving down, trying to identify the areas that feel tense. When you come across such an area, contract the muscles, hold for a count of ten, and then release. Work down your body until you feel thoroughly relaxed, from head to toe. Enjoy your bath for at least 30 minutes, topping off with more warm water as needed.

Relaxing Bath Blend

1 ounce carrier oil (such as sweet
   almond, grape seed, or jojoba)
7 drops lavender essential oil
5 drops chamomile essential oil
3 drops clary sage essential oil

THE PLANT THAT LAUNCHED AROMATHERAPY

Although essential oils have been used since biblical times, modern aromatherapy owes its origin directly to lavender. In 1928, a French chemist named René Maurice Gattefosse burned his hand in his laboratory and instinctively plunged it into the nearest vat of cool liquid—pure lavender essential oil. To the chemist's astonishment, the wound healed more quickly than normal and with no scarring. This discovery prompted Gattefosse to devote the rest of his life to studying the therapeutic uses of lavender and other essential oils.

Read Your Labels

Not all lavender is created equal. The popularity of this plant means that the market is flooded with a plethora of lavender products. All smell lovely, but if you're interested in aromatherapy benefits, most experts suggest seeking out essential oil distilled from *Lavandula angustifolia* or other high-quality French lavender.

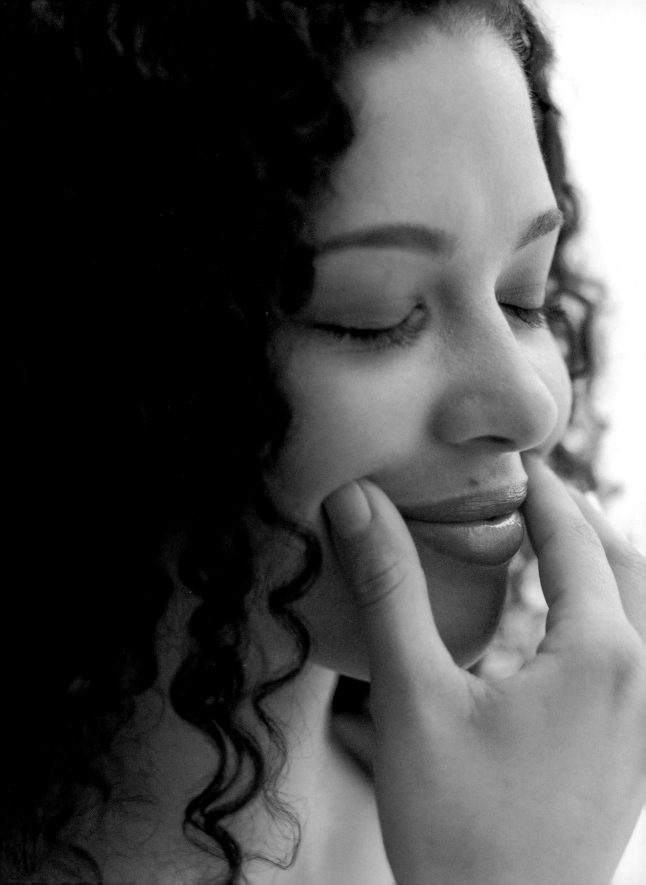

mona lisa smile

Consciously altering your expression can change how
you feel. Here's a classic exercise designed to bring
a smile to your face and lighten your mood.

From East to West, the smile is seen as an important tool to relieve
stress, depression, and self-doubt. It helps you connect with your
core of happiness and reminds you not to take things too seriously.

To lift your spirits, close your eyes and smile slightly. Breathing
deeply, place your thumb and index finger onto the corners of your
mouth and gently push them up a little further. Feel the tension ease
from your forehead. Imagine waves of joyful energy emanating from
your smile and washing over your body. If there's a part of your body
that you can tell is particularly tight or in distress, concentrate on
sending the positive energy there. Release and repeat for ten or so
smiles, until you begin to feel like da Vinci's serene lady.

Once you get used to how your body reacts when you smile in this
fashion, you can achieve much of that same feeling without even
changing your outward appearance (see the box below). This can
come in handy if you're sitting in a long business meeting, dealing
with a difficult person, or engaged in another situation in which it
might be inappropriate to break into a beaming expression.

Another Reason to Smile

We primarily use five pairs of facial
muscles to produce a smile, and
sometimes many of the 53 muscles
in our face are engaged, especially
when we flash a big grin or widen
our eyes in delight. However, even
a slight frown requires using more
muscles than a basic smile, and
chronic frowning can create deep
furrows across the forehead.

RELEASING YOUR INNER MONA LISA

With practice, you can learn to achieve that Mona Lisa feeling
without actually smiling. Begin by creating an innocuous "physical
prompt" that you can link to your Mona Lisa smile, such as putting
your thumb and forefinger together. Do this physical prompt while
practicing your smile; after a while, your body will actually associate
contented feelings with this action. Then, when you need to lighten
your spirits but it's not appropriate to break into a big grin, simply
do your physical prompt to trigger the same warm sensations.

deep-retreat massage

Sometimes you need a little help to truly unwind. Ask your partner to ease away your daytime worries with these massage techniques before you drift off to sleep.

Connect with the Cradle Rock
To thank your partner for treating you to the massage techniques at right, lie on the bed together and snuggle up behind him, resting one hand on his abdomen between his navel and ribs. Then gently rock your bodies backwards and forwards. This position not only feels comforting, it also stimulates the solar plexus chakra (see page 244 ►), creating a deep and peaceful sense of connection between the two of you.

1 Start with a relaxing back scratch; the superficial nerves on the skin's surface love to be stimulated, even at bedtime. With your partner sitting up or lying on her stomach, gently scratch all over her back. Continue on the arms, too, if they aren't too ticklish.

2 Gentle swaying motions can be profoundly relaxing. As she lies on her back with her head in your lap, hold her hand and lift her arm to a comfortable height. For a minute or so, swing her arm from side to side, varying both speed and angles to encourage the release of tension. Repeat on her other arm.

3 Stroke her forehead with alternating hands for several minutes. Asian massage practitioners believe that this particular stroke helps release a buildup of excess energy in the head.

4 Finish this deep-retreat massage with a practice used by traditional healers: Put one of your hands over the other, and rest them both on her heart. Ask her to close her eyes and take ten deep, slow breaths. (Also see "Healing Hands" on page 208 ►.)

RUBBING OUT WORRIES

Massages may seem as if they melt away the cares of the world, but do they actually counteract the physical symptoms of stress? The answer is a resounding yes. In dozens of worldwide studies, researchers found that massage can help reduce anxiety, slow respiratory and heart rates, alleviate depression, soothe tension-related headaches and eyestrain, reduce blood pressure, encourage the production of endorphins, and improve alertness on the job.

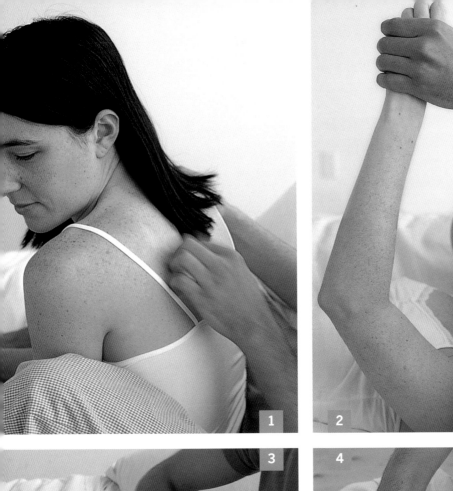

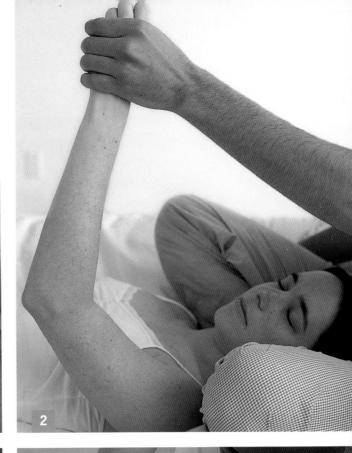

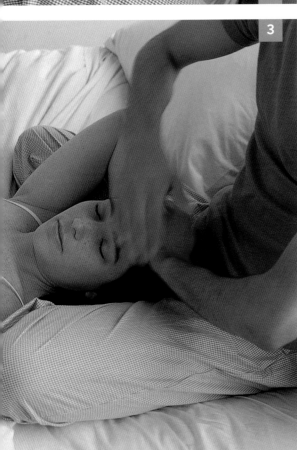

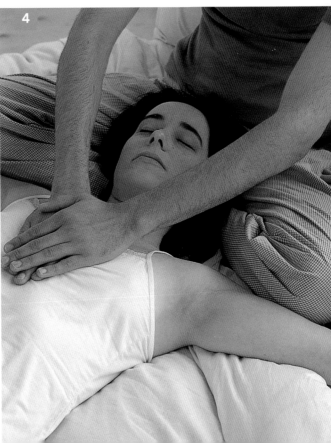

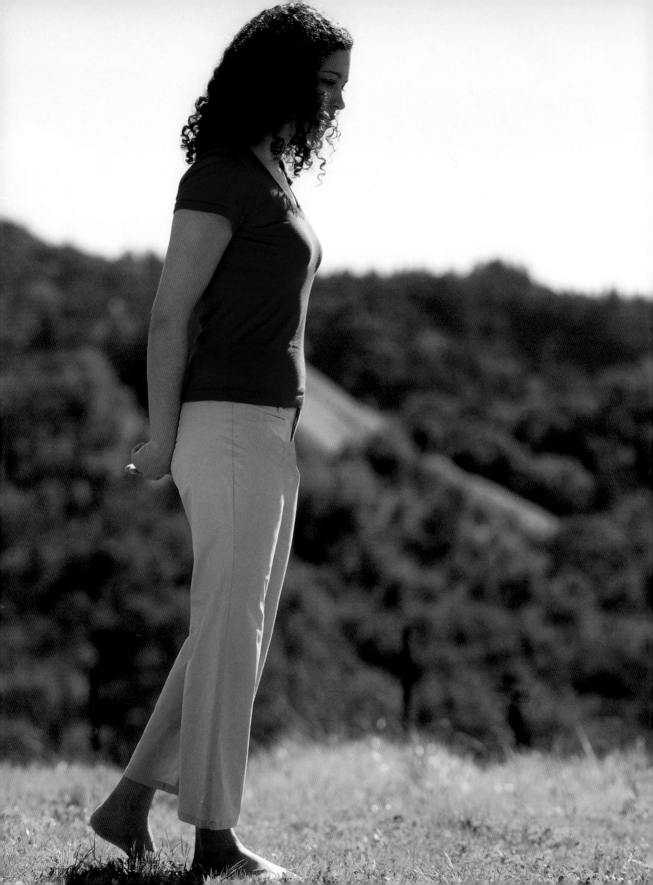

walking meditation

Practiced alone or in a group, walking can be a form
of meditation. Use the sensation of motion to focus
your thoughts and to experience your body intensely.

To begin, hold your hands in any comfortable, consistent manner:
loose at your sides, clasped behind your back, or in the prayer
position at your heart. Be aware of your feet touching the earth
and how the muscles in your body subtly work to keep you upright.

Start walking slowly, putting your feet down heel–toe, heel–toe. Keep
your eyes open but lowered, and empty your mind of all thoughts
except the sensation of moving. Feel your feet hitting the earth and
then rising again. Try to keep your muscles relaxed, releasing any
tension or tightness as you move along. Let your mind travel up
your body as you walk, registering how each part contributes to the
flowing motion. If you like, synchronize each step with a breath or
repetition of a mantra. (A mantra can be any positive or uplifting
word or phrase that has special significance for you.)

Try walking this way for about 20 to 30 minutes. When you're ready
to end the meditation, just stop naturally and stand in that spot for a
moment. Take a few deep breaths, notice how it feels to be still rather
than moving, and feel your weight resting on the earth, all of which
should contribute to your overall feeling of peacefulness.

Practitioners often prefer to walk along a loop path, but any path
is fine for this purpose. Many people also like to practice this walking
meditation technique in a group in which one person determines
the route and the pace, freeing the rest to simply concentrate on
meditating in silence. Just be sure to keep two to three feet away
from the people ahead of and behind you so they won't be distracted
by you (and, of course, to avoid bumping into one another).

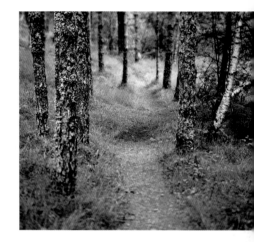

The Path to Peace
At first, walking meditation is best done
on a nature path or in a place free from
annoying distractions such as traffic, loud
noises, and crowds (but be sure to avoid
isolated areas where safety would be a
concern). Once you get more accomplished,
you might be able to mentally block out
extraneous noise so successfully that you
can practice the art of walking meditation
anywhere—even on busy city streets.

child pose

This well-known yoga pose imparts the sensation of curling up and retreating from the world. It also gently stretches your neck, back, hips, and ankles.

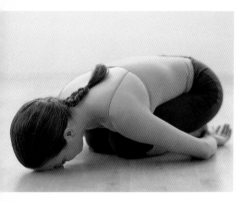

A Healthy Stretch

For the basic (not extended) Child pose, extend your hands toward your feet with your palms facing up. This is an excellent yoga position to use if you need to rest between other poses. But even if you're not yet a practiced yogi, you can use this pose to relax tension in your lower back, hips, and neck after a hard day or to unwind after vigorous exercise. Breathe deeply and quiet your thoughts as you rest.

From a kneeling position, sit back on your heels. Then lean forward and bring your chest toward your knees and your forehead toward the floor. If your forehead does not naturally come to rest on the floor, you may let your head hang or rest it on a rolled-up towel or firm pillow. Or, if you have trouble sitting on your heels, place a rolled-up towel between the back of your thighs and your calves.

To do the extended Child pose (pictured at right), stretch your arms in front of you, shoulder-width apart and with your elbows softly bent. Reach forward with your fingertips and press down your buttocks. Gently push your palms against the floor to help you sit closer to your heels. Relax your muscles, breathe deeply, and try to quiet your thoughts for at least a minute or two. To move into the basic Child pose (pictured at left), keep your head down and move your hands alongside your feet, palms facing up.

THE SPIRITUAL SIDE OF THE CHILD

While Westerners might see *Balasana* (Sanskrit for "child" and "pose") as a good stretch, yogis in India believe the position has more profound benefits. At its heart, the pose is a *pranam*, or bow, a gesture of humbleness and devotion. Many Westerners recoil at the idea of humbling themselves before anyone, but in Eastern religions the prostration is seen as a heartfelt acknowledgment of the presence of divinity and its ability to dissolve the mind's attachment to judging and criticizing others. The inward focus helps the practitioner connect with her heart, the arms stretch forward in an offering to God, and both body and mind rest in a position that can be seen as the embodiment of prayer. As such, this pose offers a retreat from the hustle and bustle of the external world.

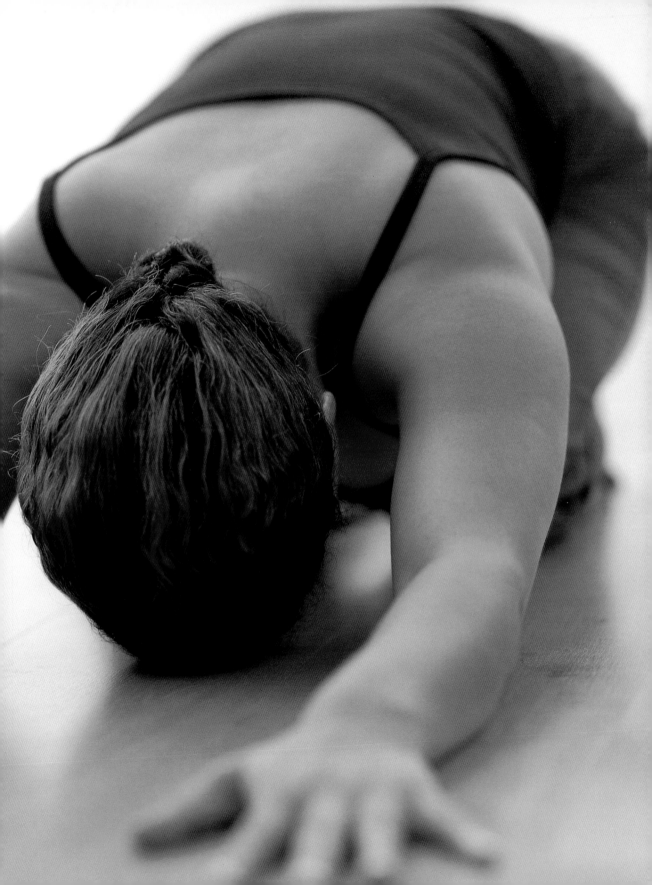

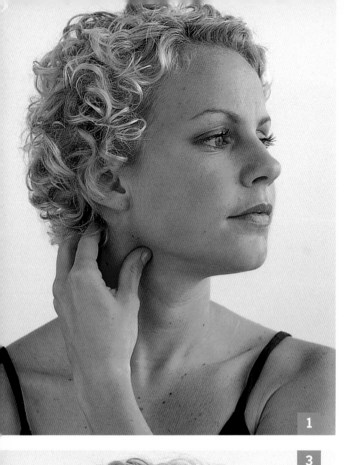

1

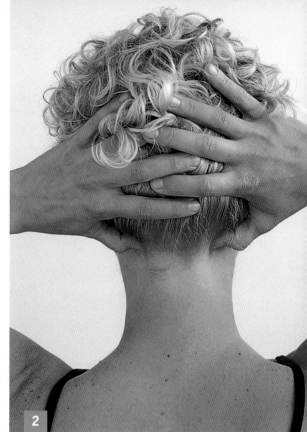

4

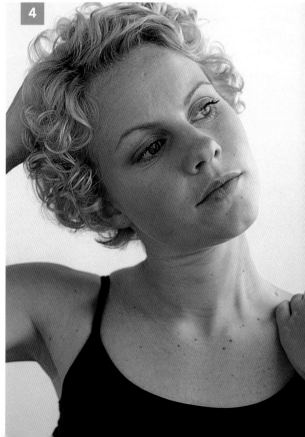

3

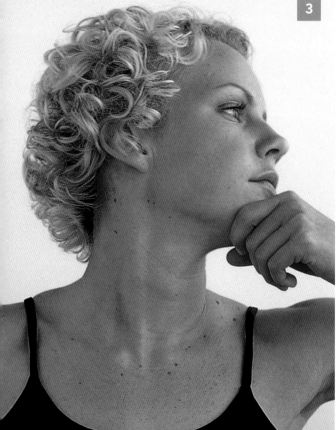

2

neck stretches

Even if no one is around to lend a helping hand, you can find some welcome neck relief with this series of do-it-yourself rubs and stretches.

1 Turn your head to the side to find your sternocleidomastoid muscle (for obvious reasons, usually just referred to as the SCM). The SCM starts on the breastbone and collarbone, crosses the neck at an angle, and attaches to the base of the skull behind the ear. Press in with your thumb and grasp the bottom of the SCM from behind. Hold using firm pressure while you slowly turn your head from side to side three times. Then repeat in a new spot one inch higher. Work both sides of your neck from bottom to top.

2 Now turn your attention to the back of your head. Press in firmly with your thumbs at the base of your skull and move them in tight, firm circles. Begin on either side of the spine and work outward along the base of your skull toward the ears. If you encounter sore points, stop and press firmly on each as you take three deep breaths.

3 Grasp something stable, such as a tabletop, with your right hand and turn your head as far to the left as is comfortable, sitting or standing up tall. Stretch your neck muscles by gently guiding your chin farther to the left with your left hand. Hold the stretch for three deep breaths. Gently release and repeat on the other side.

4 Now place your left hand on your left shoulder. With your right hand, gently guide your head down toward your right shoulder—do not use heavy pressure or you could injure your neck. Breathe in and out slowly, feeling your neck muscles gradually lengthen over the span of three breaths. Bring your head slowly back to center. Repeat on the other side. If you like, you can do this stretch a number of times, holding your head at different angles to isolate various muscles.

When Stress Is a Pain in the Neck
Ever wonder why your neck and shoulders begin to ache when you're under stress? Part of the reason seems to lie in the fight-or-flight mode that the body automatically assumes when exposed to any form of threat, whether it's a hungry tiger or a peevish boss. Many parts of the body are involved in this complicated and primitive self-preservation mechanism, including the shoulders, which hunch forward, perhaps to help us appear smaller or better protect internal organs such as the heart and lungs. The neck also gets into the act as we instinctively cock our heads forward, the better to take in external stimuli. If the stress is prolonged, holding these positions over time can result in stiff and sore muscles.

repulse monkey

When the world gets to be too much, graceful tai chi movements can help restore a sense of balance. Take a step back with Repulse Monkey—literally and figuratively.

Tactical Retreats

We often think the way to win a fight is to attack. But in tai chi, the idea of yielding (or *yin*) is as important as thrusting forward (or *yang*; see page 82 ◄). Tai chi emphasizes the ability to adapt and respond to an opponent's actions, and sometimes retreating is more powerful than resisting, attacking, or otherwise trying to win—and that's the case whether you're in a verbal argument or hand-to-hand combat.

1 Start by stepping out with your left leg, with your arms held rounded in front of you as if holding a large ball. The right arm is down, with the palm facing up; the left arm is up, with the palm facing down. Sink down, keeping your tailbone tucked in and your head up, so you create a long line from the crown of your head to the bottom of your torso. Lift your left heel and point your toes down. Concentrate your weight on your back leg; in tai chi terms, your right leg will feel "full," while your left feels "empty."

2 Step backward with your left foot. At the same time, bring your left hand around and down and your right hand around and up.

3 End with your left hand down by your belly button, palm turned up, and your right hand reaching out in front of you, at about ear level, fingers pointing to the sky, palm facing down. Your right leg is now extended in front and feeling empty, toes are down, heel is up; your left leg should feel full. Repeat Steps 1 through 3 on the other side (step back with your right leg, with the left arm down and the right up). Do two to four times each, alternating right and left sides.

MEDITATION IN MOTION

For Westerners accustomed to a bombardment of external stimuli, it isn't always easy to quiet the mind and gain full awareness of the body. Yet even for folks who are easily distracted during sitting meditation, tai chi can provide a form of moving meditation that's more engaging and effective. The emphasis on slow, controlled movements, inward focus, and proper body alignment compels the practitioner to concentrate and be fully present in the moment.

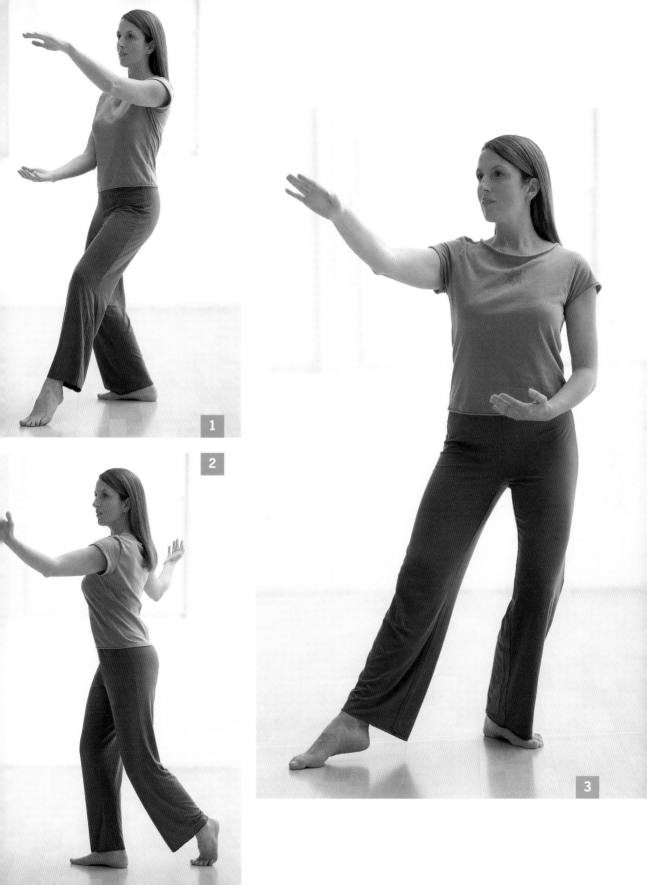

1

2

3

comfort

Reading a book, eating certain foods, even sticking to a bedtime routine. Comfort means different things to different people, but it always involves simple pleasures that bring a sense of quiet contentment.

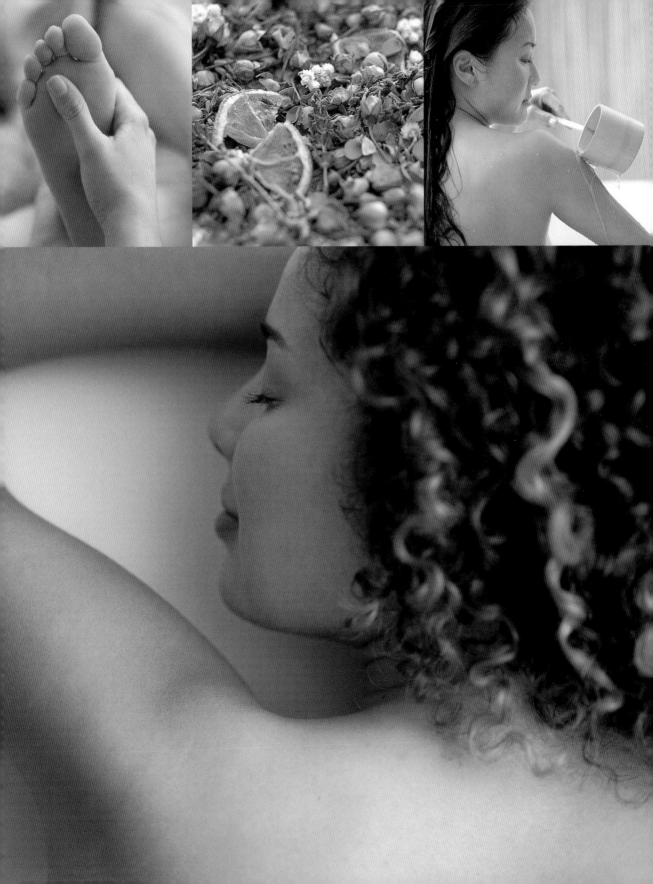

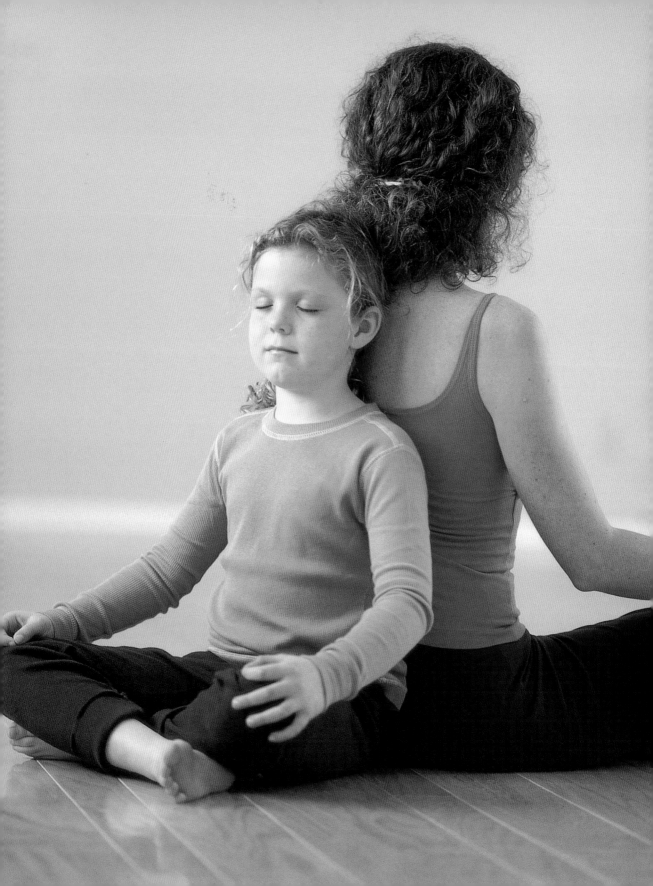

comfort

We all have our own notions of comfort. For one woman, it's slipping into a pair of ratty pajamas that others would immediately consign to the rag bin. For another, it's digging into an admittedly odd dish that somehow has been a favorite family recipe for six generations. Many people feel deeply comforted when they surround themselves with family and friends, while others find solace in a solitary walk or an evening spent alone reading in a well-worn easy chair.

Our paths might be different, but the end is the same: Comfort involves quieting the mind, feeding the soul, and draining tension from the body. It restores a sense of hope and soothes away the worries of the day (or at least puts them into perspective). And, unlike simple relaxation, it includes a sense of connection—to happy past times, to beloved people, or just to one's own old, best self.

The activities in this chapter provide many avenues for seeking comfort—physically demanding ones, such as yoga and tai chi, as well as more passive pursuits, such as meditation and aromatherapy. As you peruse them, they're also bound to remind you of your own sources of personal comfort, the things, activities, and people you can turn to when you're in need of a little TLC.

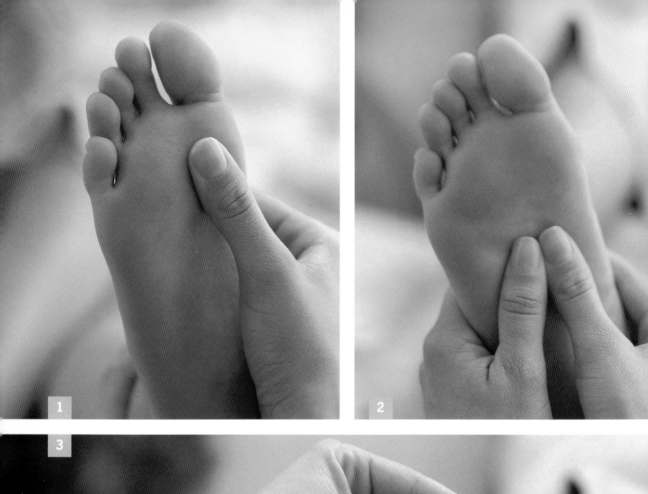

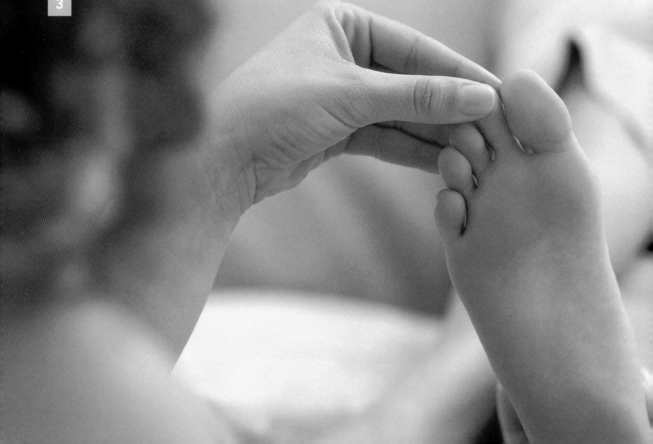

foot reflexology

Reflexologists believe feet have zones that when pressed exert beneficial influences on other body parts. A foot massage also ranks high among life's simple pleasures.

Foot massages really are wonderful at melting away tension, and the reflexology techniques employed here add a new dimension of health benefits to this treatment. (Also see page 44 ◄ for a reflexology map of the hand.) Recruit a friend to treat you to these soothing steps:

1 Get into a comfortable position for massaging your friend's foot. To activate the reflexology zones, begin by using your thumb to make deep, overlapping circles over the entire surface of her heel and arch. Then place your thumb just above her arch at the base of the ball of the foot and press into one of the grooves between the bones that lead up to the toes. Circle with your thumb up each groove, moving from the top of the arch toward each toe.

2 Grip the foot with both hands, with thumbs holding the bottom of the foot at mid-heel level. With your thumbs braced side by side for firm pressure, glide up the sole to the grooves in the ball of the foot and then up to the space between the big and second toes. Ease your grip and slide lightly back to the heel. Repeat two more times.

3 Give each toe an individual massage by pressing your thumb and index finger together and circling from base to tip. Then wiggle each toe backward, forward, and around in circles, starting with small circles and spiraling into bigger ones, being careful not to bend the toes too far. For a soothing finish, do a foot sweep: Contour and press your hands together on the top and bottom of your friend's foot. Gently pull your hands toward you and off her toes three times. Then repeat all these massage steps on the other foot.

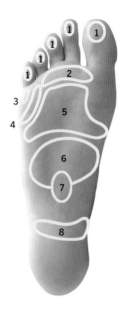

Right Foot Reflexology Map
Here are some of the key reflexology points on the sole of your right foot:

1 Sinus, head, and brain
2 Eyes and ears
3 Arms
4 Shoulders
5 Lungs and breasts
6 Liver
7 Kidneys
8 Sciatic nerve

rock the baby

Releasing tense hip joints with this yoga pose soothes and stretches your back. Dissipating the physical tension can offer surprising emotional rewards as well.

A Rush of Emotions

In some yoga traditions, the hips are considered the seat of emotional vulnerability. This means that as you release physical tension in this area, you also might experience the release of pent-up emotions, such as fear, anger, or sorrow. That can be a bit unsettling, but if you let these feelings rise, wash over you, and pass, you'll appreciate the relief that comes with detaching from emotions (rather than clinging to them), as well as the clarity that comes from releasing them.

Sit with both your legs extended in front of you. Bend your right knee and lift your right leg toward your chest. Keeping your back as straight as possible, hug your leg inward and gently rock it from side to side, the same way you'd rock a baby. Ideally, your elbows will wrap around your knee and foot, but use any grasp that feels comfortable to you. As you rock, take four to eight deep breaths, and then repeat the *asana,* or pose, with your other leg.

While you're doing this or other poses that stretch the hips, focus on your second *chakra*—one of seven spots in the body where yogis believe that channels of energy intersect (see page 244 ▶ for a chart and more information on chakras). The second chakra, which is located just below the navel, is thought to govern creativity, sexuality, fertility, and sensuality, as well as emotions such as anger, fear, and the instinct to nurture. Yogis believe that the second chakra, when well balanced (that is, not blocked or overactive), can help women feel more powerful, creative, and sensual.

FLEXIBLE HIPS CAN HELP YOUR BACK

We all know that poor posture, incorrect lifting techniques, and sedentary lifestyles can contribute to lower back pain. What few of us realize, however, is that sometimes those back problems actually are rooted in the hips. That's because chronic sitting (in your car or at your desk, for instance) can result in shortened hip flexors—the muscles at the front of your hips. Even certain exercises, such as leg lifts, stair climbing, and bicycling, can tighten the hip flexors. Stretching the hip flexors and working on maintaining a full range of motion in the hips will help avoid these problems.

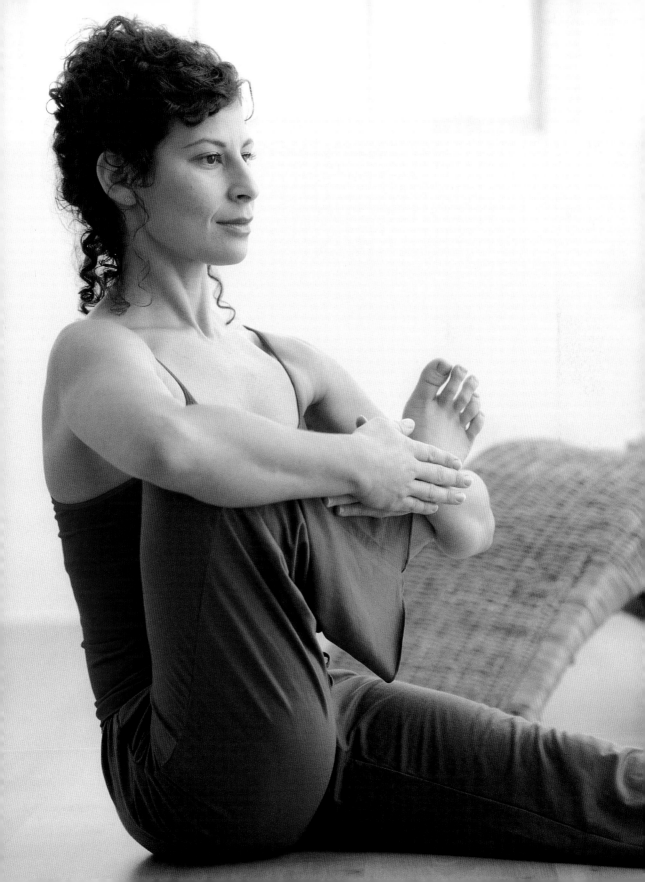

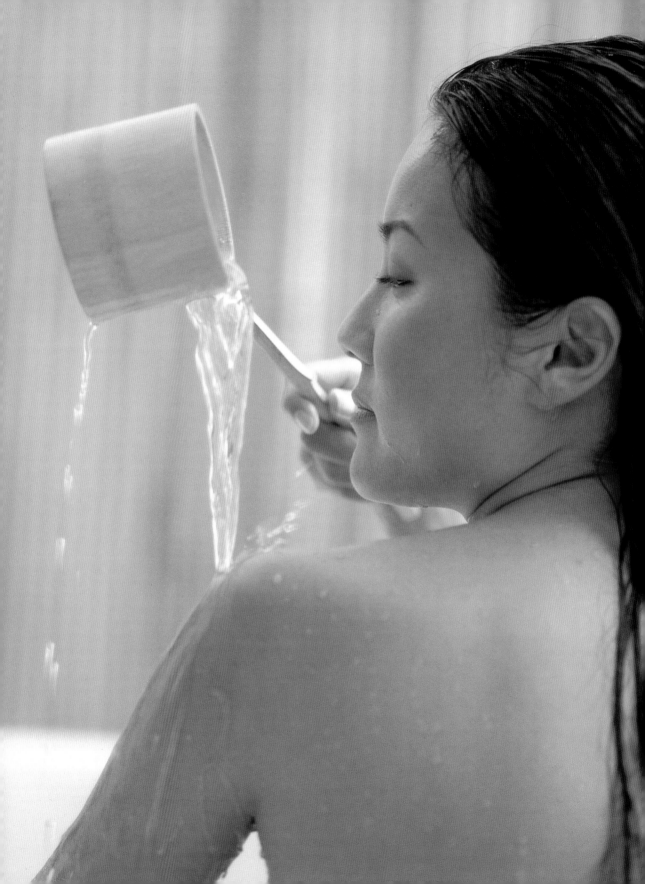

bath therapy

When it comes to providing a respite from everyday cares, few things are more satisfying than a bath, especially when you use a ladle to caress your body with fragrant water.

Draw a very warm bath—not scalding, mind you, but hot enough that you will have to ease into the water slowly. After the tub fills, add a blend of essential oils specially chosen for their comforting qualities (see the chamomile-lavender recipe at right, which will also help moisturize your skin). Before you enter the tub, stir the water with your hands to thoroughly mix the essential oils.

Get into the tub, and spend a few minutes just soaking in the warm water. Close your eyes and take deep, cleansing breaths. Then, using a ladle, pour warm bathwater over your shoulders and the middle of your back. Notice how the water soothes your muscles and helps calm your mind. Slowly ladle water onto the top and back of your head, being careful not to let it run over your face (those essential oils won't feel very good if they get in your eyes). Ladle bathwater onto the tops of your arms. Keep ladling slowly and methodically as a form of meditation, visualizing the water washing away your worries. When you've finished, lie back, close your eyes, and soak for another ten minutes or so, remaining in a peaceful, meditative state.

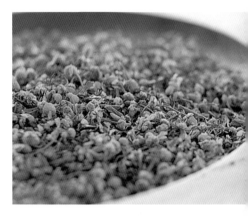

Comforting Bath Blend

1 teaspoon sweet almond carrier oil

3 drops chamomile essential oil

3 drops lavender essential oil

2 drops geranium essential oil

A GUIDE TO BATH PRODUCTS

Bath salts typically are made from sea salt and essential oils or other fragrances; they help soften the skin and reputedly draw toxins from the body. *Bath foams* create bubbles, release pleasant scents, and can serve as a substitute for soap. *Bath oils,* which generally contain essential oils or other fragrances suspended in a light carrier oil, moisturize your skin. *Bath* (or *shower*) *gels* are a kind of liquid soap. *Bath teas* are tea bags filled with dried herbs purported to have a variety of therapeutic effects when left to steep in bathwater.

Calming Chamomile

When drunk as a tea, chamomile (either the Roman or German type) is said to relax the body and induce sleep; it also can help settle an upset stomach. As an essential oil, the herb (pictured above) is often used to alleviate insomnia and nervousness. Its anti-inflammatory properties can also help soothe irritated or sunburned skin.

pleasures of potpourri

A perennial aromatherapy favorite, lovely bags or bowls of delicious scents can spice up a room, sweeten a friendship, or even evoke memories and moods.

Potpourri is a combination of aromatic and decorative ingredients, such as dried flower petals, leaves, fruits, spices, and wood shavings, sprinkled with essential oils. Better-quality potpourri also contains fixatives, such as orrisroot, that absorb and slowly release the essential oils, helping the fragrance last longer. You can purchase ready-made potpourri at gift and craft stores, but you might find it even more rewarding to create your own special blend.

First, find a potpourri recipe that sounds appealing; look in books, browse online, or try the recipe at left. Craft shops, herb catalogs, and natural food stores will have the ingredients you need (as might your own backyard), but you'll also need a few tools, such as clean glass jars, a kitchen scale (for measuring ingredients), and glass eyedroppers (one for each oil you use). Be forewarned: Making potpourri doesn't take much time, but the mix has to settle for about three weeks before it's ready to use, so plan ahead if you're making gifts.

Once your mixture is ready, you can put it in pretty bowls and place them strategically throughout your home (avoid using very strongly scented potpourri where you're eating, however, because it can interfere with the taste of your food). You also can make sachets by placing potpourri in small bags of porous cloth, such as linen, cotton, or silk, tied with ribbons; these impart a delicate scent to your clothes when placed in closets or dresser drawers. If you really want to unleash the aroma of your mixture, sprinkle the potpourri in a pot of water and simmer it on the stove. Besides these purely atmospheric uses, potpourri can serve practical purposes: Ingredients such as rosemary, sage, cedar, citronella, and lavender help repel moths, for example, while a mixture of chamomile, bergamot, lavender, and clary sage, placed at your bedside, helps promote a good night's sleep.

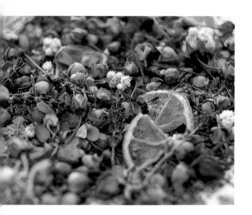

Peaceful Potpourri
Make a comforting potpourri from a mixture of dried orange rinds and lavender, rose, and jasmine petals—perfect beside your favorite reading chair, on your nightstand, or on your desk. A few drops of the corresponding essential oils will make the fragrance more pronounced and longer-lasting.

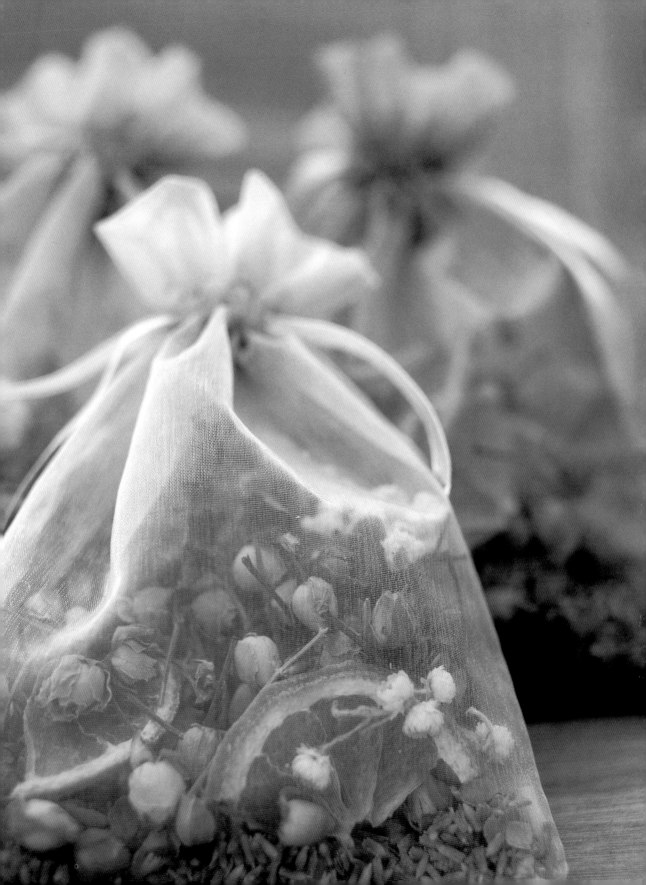

comfort

energy holds

Inspired by Ayurvedic chakra work and other ancient forms of healing, these moves let a friend or your partner use the power of touch to connect.

Healing Hands

Many energy healers believe that we have a slightly positive charge in our right hand and a slightly negative charge in our left hand. When we touch someone with both hands, the difference in charges is supposed to cause a mild but potent electrical current to flow between the hands. This current can help break up any energy blockages in the person we're touching, allowing his or her own energy to flow freely and helping to restore balance, health, and wellbeing.

Find a willing partner to treat you to these comforting energy holds by following the directions in these four simple steps:

1 Briskly rub your hands together for about 20 seconds to help warm them. Place your hands under your friend's head, with your thumbs above her ears and the rest of your fingers beneath. Don't press down; just hold her head lightly for a minute or so to help her relax as she lies comfortably on her back.

2 Rest your right hand below her navel and your left hand on her forehead. Keeping your left hand still, rock your right hand from side to side, using enough pressure to gently rock her hips from side to side. Rock her for 20 seconds or so, then rest for 20 seconds, keeping your hands in place. Alternate rocking and resting for a few minutes.

3 Have your friend roll over onto her stomach. Place one hand on the top of her tailbone and your other hand at the base of her neck (corresponding to the second and fifth chakras respectively; see page 244 ▶ for more details on chakras). Rock her hips from side to side with your lower hand for 20 seconds; then be still for 20 seconds, always keeping both of your hands in place. Repeat this cycle for a few minutes until her breathing becomes deep, calm, and regular.

4 Place one of your hands over the other and hold them a few inches above her lower back for a moment. (You're tapping into the energy field that many traditional healers believe radiates from the body; see "Healing Hands" at left.) Then set your hands lightly on her back and rock gently, alternating between rocking and stillness. Be sensitive to any sense of warmth or tingling—signs of pent-up energy being released. After five full breaths, slowly lift your hands, and hold them a few inches above her body for another moment.

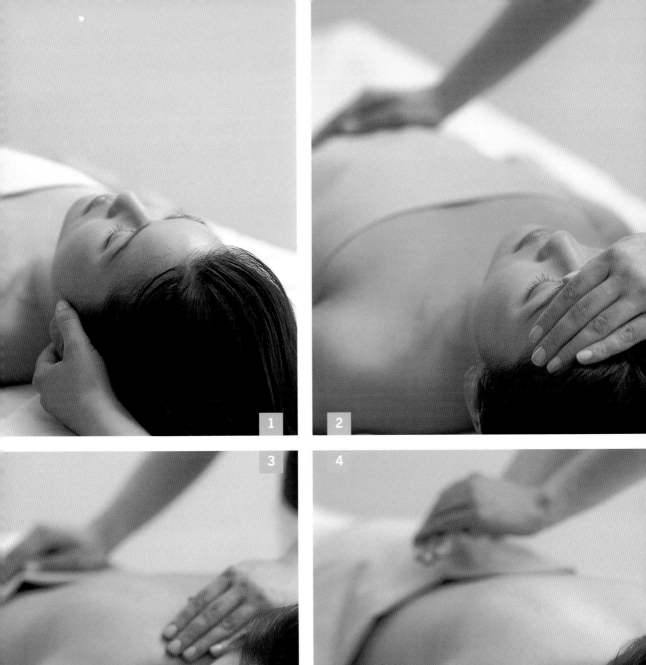

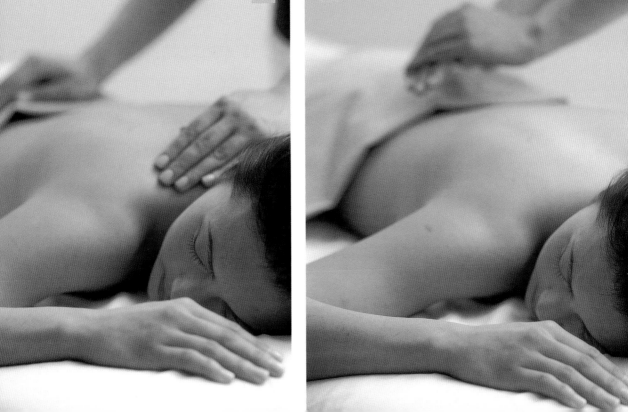

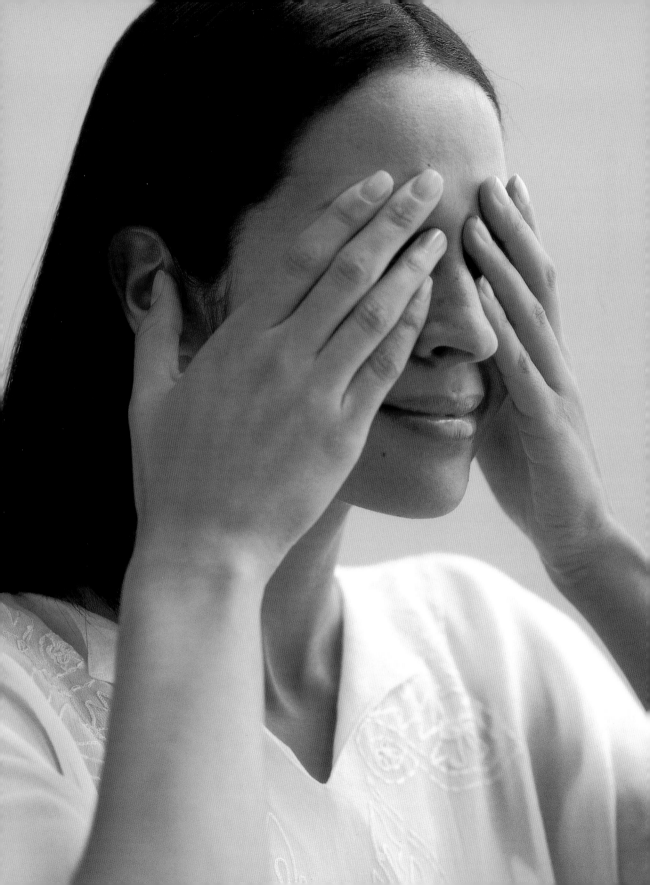

humming bee breath

The pleasing, audible vibration in this yoga breathing practice helps to clarify the mind and calm the spirit. Easy to do, it can be enjoyed by children and adults.

Called the *bhramari pranayama* in Sanskrit, the Humming Bee Breath can help you with your meditation, as well as help relieve tension, dispel anger, lower blood pressure, soothe insomnia, and inspire an "indescribable bliss in the hearts of yogis," according to the classic manual on yoga, the *Hatha Yoga Pradipika,* written by a 15th-century Indian yogi. It is a wonderful exercise for those times when you need to calm yourself—or a small child (or both).

Sit in a comfortable meditation pose, with your back straight. Place your hands over your eyes. Use your thumbs to press down gently on the tragi, the little flaps at the front of your ears, so they seal off the openings to the ear canals. (The idea is to cut off external sensory inputs.) Inhale deeply. Then exhale slowly through your nostrils, while humming high in the back of your mouth, so you feel a vibration on your soft palate (the soft, fleshy back part of the roof of your mouth). Draw out each exhalation as long as you can. Practice for three to seven breaths; then release, close your eyes, rest your hands on your knees, and enjoy the quiet space you have created.

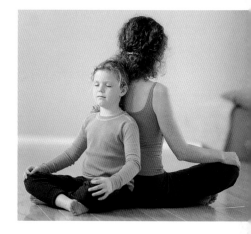

The Virtues of Quiet Time
Sharing peaceful moments with children can promote deeper bonding and greater physical and emotional awareness. To help rein in a child's naturally jumpy mind, as you practice yoga breathing together, try counting aloud or talking periodically to find out how your child is feeling.

YOGA AND CHILDREN

By practicing yoga, children as young as four years old can learn to be more aware of their bodies and emotions, to relax more easily, and to cultivate mental focus. It also helps them develop better coordination, posture, and balance. Some children learn yoga for medical reasons—to deal with chronic pain or help alleviate asthma symptoms, for example. When enrolling your child in a class, be sure the instructor has training in children's yoga: doing too-challenging poses can damage a child's growing body (and self-esteem).

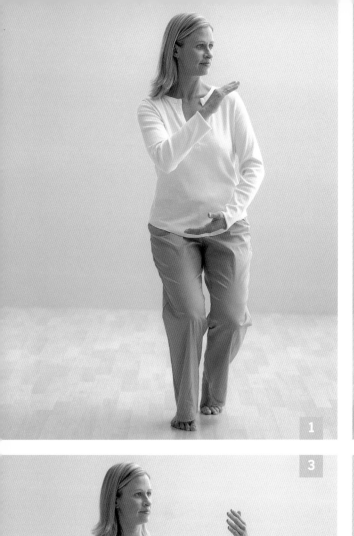

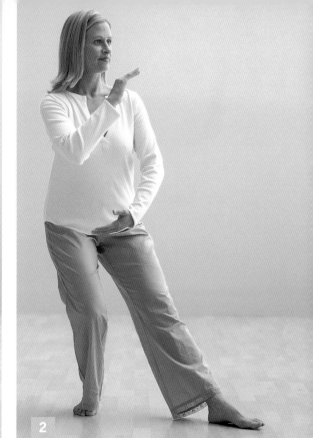

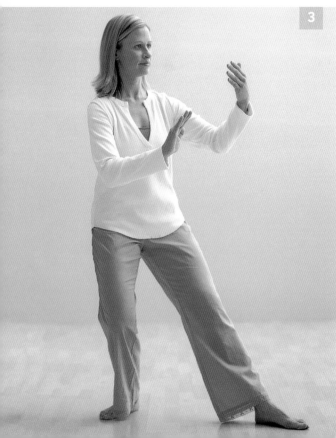

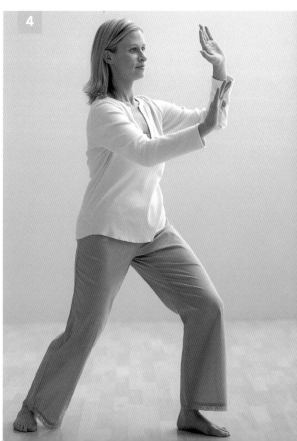

works at shuttles

The balanced, embracing motions of Fair Lady Works at Shuttles, which honors women's handiwork and service, make this tai chi movement a soothing exercise.

1 Stand with your left foot behind your right foot, knees slightly bent and positioned directly over your toes. Lift your right arm across your body to about shoulder height, with the elbow bent and the palm facing down. Bring your left arm down below your belly button, keeping the elbow bent and the palm up. Keep your elbows, wrists, and knees soft; that is, don't form any hard angles at the joints.

2 Step out with your left foot, sinking your weight onto the right foot. Keep your arms round, with the right hand still above the left.

3 Roll your hips back as you move your left arm up (with the palm now facing in). Draw your right arm back, palm now facing out.

4 Push both hands out in front of you until the left arm is above your right arm and the fingers are tipped slightly back. Shift your weight to follow the hands' movements and bend your left knee. Repeat Steps 1 through 4 three more times.

My Fair Lady
The formal name of this tai chi movement (Fair Lady Works at Shuttles) comes from the ancient Chinese belief that the world is square and that the heavens are supported by a tortoise's four legs, which also represent the four points of the compass. According to Chinese legend, a loyal serving maid weaves tirelessly at four looms belonging to the Taoist immortals, moving in turn from shuttle to shuttle—hence these movements traditionally are repeated four times in different directions.

WHO'S PRACTICING TAI CHI?

Most of the world's tai chi practitioners live in China. In fact, Dennis Kelly, founder of Tai Chi–USA, claims there are more people doing tai chi in China on any given day than there are people doing all other kinds of exercises, combined, around the world. In Western countries, the majority of tai chi practitioners are women, mainly because many men think of it as a "soft" exercise that neither builds muscles nor gives the cardiovascular system enough of a workout. But, increasingly, male athletes—including football players and Olympic-level sled-racers—are turning to tai chi both to develop mental control and to learn to stay calm under pressure.

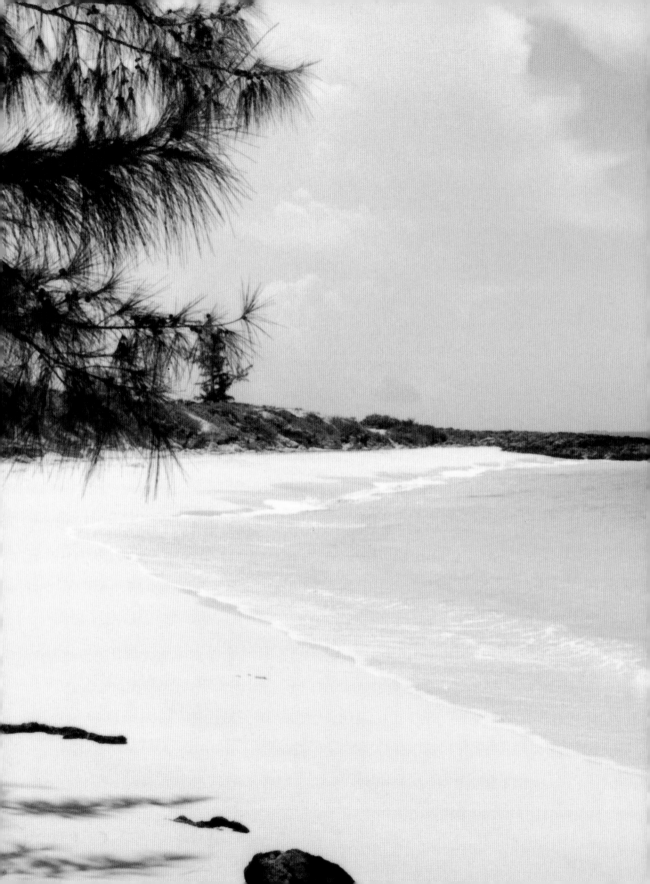

Find a place in your home or workplace where you can count on being undisturbed for ten minutes or so. Sit in a comfortable, straight-backed chair, and rest your forearms and hands lightly in your lap or on the arms of the chair. Close your eyes and begin breathing slowly and deeply. Push away any thoughts racing through your mind—the need to call the vet or the work project that's due next week—and just concentrate on the regular rise and fall of your breath. Start by focusing on the soles of your feet and work your way slowly up to the small muscles in your scalp, consciously relaxing your entire body and applying just enough muscle control to keep you sitting upright in your chair.

the greatest escape

Now you're ready for your great escape. Visualize your favorite setting, a beautiful place where you feel happy and totally at ease. For many people, that special venue involves the curve of a white-sand beach lapped by a serene, azure sea. Picture yourself walking along the beach. Feel the powdery sand crunching under your feet and the gentle breeze ruffling your hair. Listen to the steady rhythm of the waves, and enjoy the heady fragrance of the plumeria, ginger, and other tropical flowers that grow just beyond the sandy shores. Set your towel down on the beach and stretch out in the sunshine. After a while, walk to the sea and plunge into the bathtub-warm water. Swim contentedly until you're pleasantly tired, and then return to your towel, stretching out again on the beach and letting the breeze gradually dry off your wet body. When you're ready, stand, pick up your towel, and head for home, knowing that you can return to your solitary paradise any time you wish.

comfort

salmon with wine sauce

Serve this savory salmon dish with mashed potatoes and a medley of roasted vegetables and you'll find that healthy comfort food need not be an oxymoron.

Ingredients

1 cup dry red wine (a Merlot, Pinot Noir, or Beaujolais works best)

1 cup low-fat chicken broth

3 tablespoons red-wine vinegar

2 tablespoons minced shallots

Kosher salt and white pepper

6 tablespoons chilled unsalted butter, cut into 6 pieces

4 salmon fillets with skin, about 6 to 8 ounces each

Olive oil

• Serves: 4
• Prep time: 15 minutes
• Cook time: 40 minutes

Nutritional Information Per Serving
In general, Atlantic salmon is lower in fat than Pacific salmon.

Calories	507
Kilojoules	2,121
Protein	35 g
Carbohydrates	2.5 g
Total Fat	39 g
Saturated Fat	15 g
Cholesterol	147 mg
Sodium	261 mg
Dietary Fiber	.04 g

Back before we knew about cholesterol and heart disease, "comfort food" often consisted of such dishes as macaroni and cheese, roasted red meats, and potatoes laden with butter and cream. But now we know there's nothing comforting about the health risks posed by such foods, and the search is on for better alternatives. This dish fills that bill: Salmon is one of the darlings of the food world, beloved by chefs and cardiologists alike. Serve it with the roasted or sautéed vegetables of your choice and a judicious portion of mashed potatoes (use creamy potatoes such as Yukon golds to reduce the need for butter and moisten them with buttermilk, low-fat milk, or chicken broth). You'll have a deeply satisfying meal that's packed with vitamins, omega-3 fatty acids, and protein—comforting indeed!

1 In a small saucepan, combine the wine, chicken broth, vinegar, and shallots. Bring to a boil and cook over medium-high heat until the mixture is reduced to a half cup or so, about 25 minutes.

2 Strain the sauce through a fine mesh sieve, discarding the shallots, and return the liquid to the saucepan. Season to taste with salt and pepper. (The sauce can be made ahead of time up to this point.)

3 To finish the sauce, heat almost to the boiling point. Remove from the heat, and gradually whisk in the butter one tablespoon at a time until the sauce thickens slightly. Keep warm.

4 Preheat the grill to medium-hot. Brush the salmon fillets with olive oil and season with salt and pepper. Cook skin side down over the hottest part of the grill for six to eight minutes. Turn the fish over and cook until it is just opaque, three to four minutes longer.

5 Remove the salmon from the grill, and take off the skin. Arrange individual servings on plates and serve with the red wine sauce.

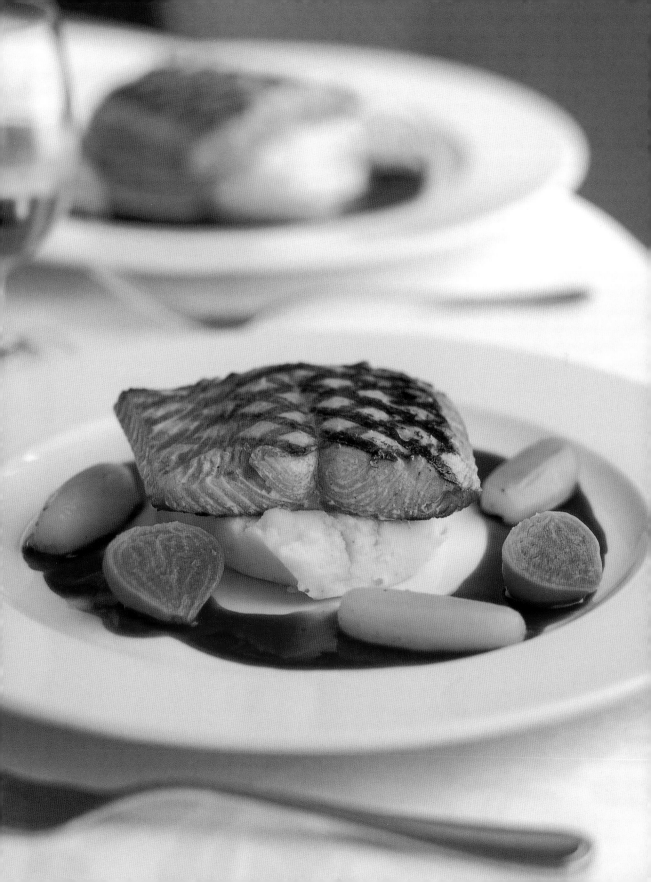

entice

The poet e. e. cummings wrote, "be of love (a little) more careful than of anything." Anyone who's been in a committed relationship knows what good advice that is—and how hard it is to follow sometimes.

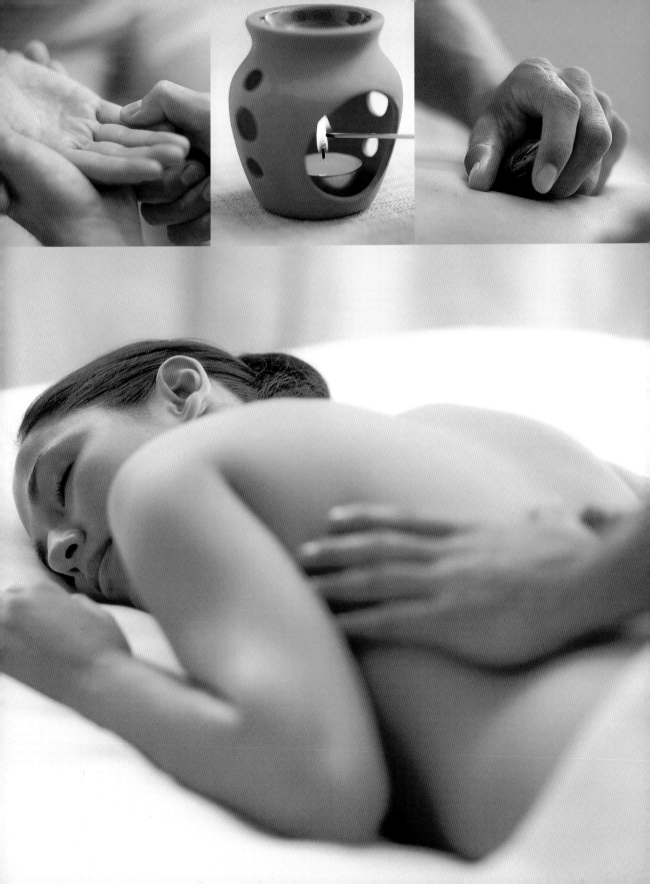

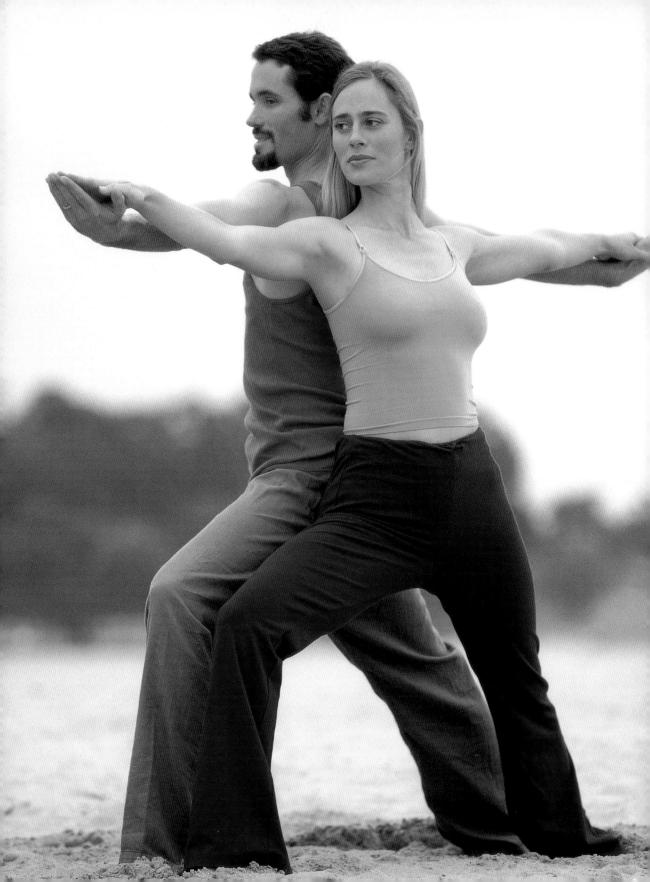

entice

Like a living organism, a loving relationship requires careful nurturing. When you are in the first blush of love, you instinctively put in the time and effort necessary to cultivate your budding romance. But many long-term couples find that romance often gets lost in the humdrum of everyday living. Your energy goes to your children, your friends, your work, your errands—and often there's precious little left over to lavish on your partner.

It doesn't have to be that way. Sometimes the smallest thoughtful gesture is enough to remind you both of the wellspring of affection that lies beneath you—a quick hug as you run out the door in the morning, a telephone call to share an inside joke in the middle of the day, a bouquet of spring wildflowers perched on the nightstand one evening. And sometimes it takes something quite out of the ordinary to spice things up: a hot stone massage, a session of shared meditation, a candlelit meal featuring (supposed) aphrodisiacs. You'll find many ideas for rekindling romance in this chapter (or, if you're unattached, maybe sparking a new one). Some are frankly sexual, others are luxuriously sensuous, and a few simply cultivate the sense of intimate connection that makes you a couple.

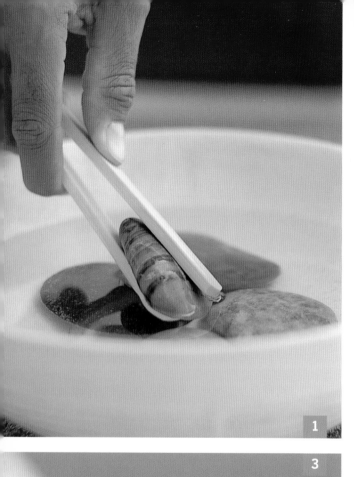

1

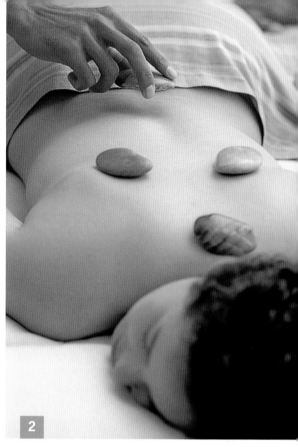

2

3

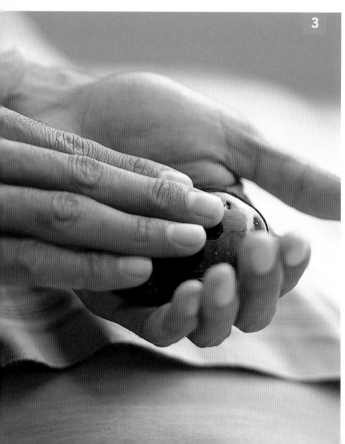

4

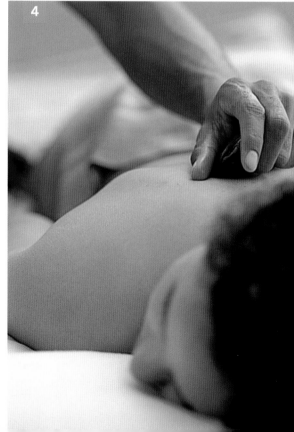

hot stones

Placed on key energy points and used as massage tools, hot stones help you and your loved one relax and give you a new way to touch each other.

Provide your partner with these massage instructions, as you prepare for your treatment by lying facedown on a bed or a comfortable mat on the floor, with your arms at your sides and palms facing up:

1 Put seven flat, smooth, clean stones in a large bowl or pan and cover them with boiling water. Heat the stones for about five to ten minutes. Using tongs, remove the stones from the hot water one at a time and dry each as you're about to place it on your partner. Test the temperature of the stones with your hand to be sure that they're not too hot. Start by placing a stone in each of your partner's palms.

2 Place one stone on the muscles next to each shoulder blade, and another stone at the base of the neck. Finish with a stone gently placed at the base of the spine. Allow your partner to rest for ten minutes, so she can feel the warmth and heft of the stones stimulate energy points and help coax away her tension.

3 Once the stones have cooled, take them away in the order in which you placed them. Then remove the remaining stone from the hot water and dry it off. Hold it in the palm of your hand and pour a little massage oil on it, rubbing the stone between your hands to cover it with the oil. For added pleasure, add three drops of essential oil to the massage oil; rose, jasmine, and ylang-ylang are soothing oils.

4 Use one of the smooth edges of the warm, oiled stone to gently massage your partner's back. Placing the stone on one side of the base of the spine (never press directly on the spine), glide it upward with light pressure in one smooth movement. Stroke up to, and then along, the inside of the right shoulder blade. Repeat this gliding stroke twice more, gradually increasing the amount of pressure but not rubbing too hard. Now repeat on the other side of the back.

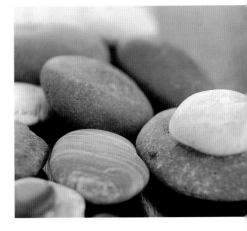

Choosing the Right Rocks
You can find rocks suitable for massage at most craft stores or collect them from a beach or riverbed. They should have a bit of weight to them but not be so heavy that they would cause discomfort when placed on your partner's body.

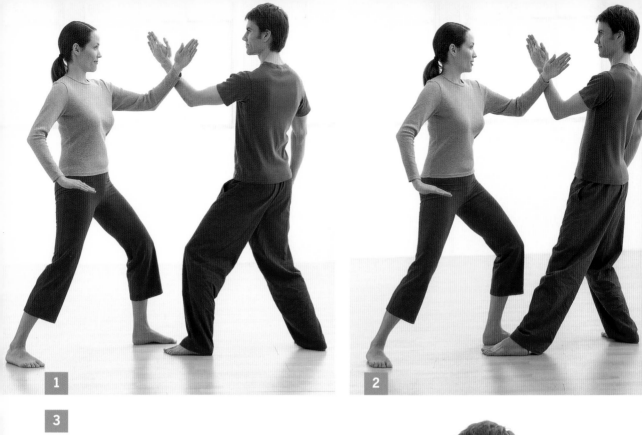

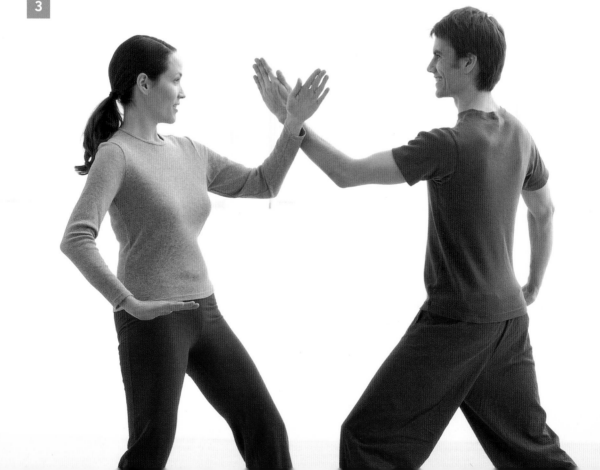

push hands

Often used as sparring practice in the martial arts, Push Hands can be a shared tai chi exercise that helps you develop greater sensitivity to each other's movements.

1 Starting an arm's distance away from your partner, step into the bow position: one leg forward and bent at the knee and one leg extended back. You both should have the same leg (that is, the right or the left) forward and feel balanced. Keep your head up and your tailbone down, so your spine is lengthened. Each of you then raises the forward arm (the arm on the same side as your forward foot) to chest height, with the elbow softly bent. Keep the palm facing away from your partner's hand and your fingers straight. Rest the back of your forearm on the back of your partner's forearm, a bit like crossed swords. Hold your other hand down and at your side, with the elbow softly bent and your fingers out straight, palm facing the ground. Remember to keep your shoulders down and relaxed.

2 Keeping your feet stationary, shift your weight forward as you gently push on your partner's forearm with your forearm. Your partner should yield to your force and shift his weight backward.

3 Next it's your partner's turn to press forward, shifting his weight toward you and exerting pressure with his forearm. This time, you respond by yielding and shifting your weight backward. Take turns with your partner—alternating pressing forward and yielding—with your feet remaining in place as your arms move back and forth in a tight, circular manner (picture the action of the wheels of a locomotive). Keep your hips loose so they can rotate freely, and absorb your partner's movements by keeping your knees bent, not by leaning back or tipping forward dramatically. Push hands in this manner for as long as you can both can stay relaxed and focused, alternating sides from time to time, if you like.

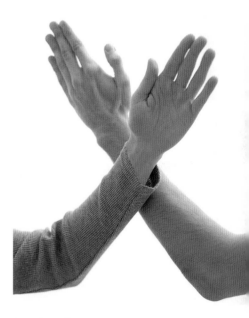

Armed and Ready

As you rock back and forth in Push Hands (Step 3), your forward hands and forearms can remain in the same position relative to each other. Or, if it feels more natural, they can travel up and down each other's arms, never going past the wrist or elbow.

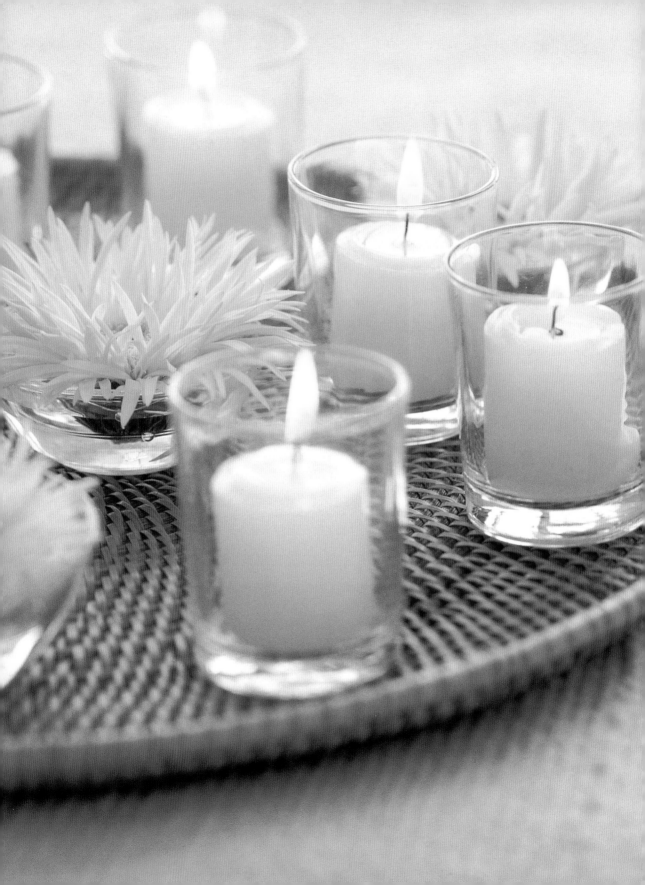

Though we are creatures of the age of technology, the soft, dancing light provided by candles still enchants us. Placing a few or even a whole collection of candles throughout a room can transform it into a lovely, magical space in just a matter of minutes: Your kitchen suddenly feels like an atmospheric small cafe, your bathroom a luxurious spa, and, perhaps most dramatically, your bedroom a mysterious and seductive hideaway.

the romance of candles

Using essential oils enhances the romantic experience. In the bedroom, you might try using a candle made with the oil from ylang-ylang flowers; not only is it reputed to be an aphrodisiac, it's supposed to alleviate performance anxieties, as does vetiver, also known as "the oil of tranquility." Candles scented with jasmine, sandalwood, neroli, patchouli, frankincense, geranium, or rose also are thought to put one in the mood for love.

Many gift and health food stores sell aromatherapy (versus standard scented) candles. You also can make your own by adding 30 to 60 drops of essential oil to eight ounces of candle wax; you'll find candle-making kits at craft stores. Or take the easy way out: Just place a few drops of essential oil on any unscented candle, near its wick. As the wax melts, the aroma will be released. (Remember that essential oils are flammable; don't use too much, and don't put them directly on a burning wick. You don't want things to get that hot in the bedroom!)

hands to hearts

When you share yoga practice with your partner, you develop a special awareness of each other's body and a state of mind that provides a peaceful way to connect.

The Chemistry of Staying Together
After the first blush of sexual attraction fades (see "The Chemistry of Attraction" below), your lingering feelings of tenderness can be attributed partly to the hormone oxytocin, which researchers have linked with emotional bonding. Longtime lovers often benefit from periodic rushes of this hormone and stress-busting endorphins. In fact, some researchers assert that couples may stay together due to a physical addiction to the very chemicals that fueled their love in the first place.

Standing face-to-face, place your right hand over your partner's heart and your left hand on his or her back. Have your partner do the same for you. Breathing slowly and deeply, gaze into each other's eyes and practice the Microcosmic Orbit: As you inhale, try to visualize light or energy gathering deep in your belly and rising to the crown of your head. As you exhale slowly, picture the energy cascading back down from your crown through your body. Then visualize this same effect taking place within your partner's body.

Hold this pose as long as you remain comfortable and connected. Feel the depth of your union, and the sense of love, trust, and contentment that passes between you. If one of you is troubled or hurting, visualize healing energy flowing from the other's body; if one of you has just had joyful news, feed the other with your happiness. Although this is not a physically demanding exercise, extended practice can be an intense form of meditation and intimacy.

THE CHEMISTRY OF ATTRACTION

Not to dampen any idealistic notions of romance, but much of the yearning and giddiness you feel when you fall in love is powered by a series of chemical reactions in the body. Reproductive hormones such as testosterone (which is produced by both men and women) prompt the search for a mate, and many scientists believe that a specialized area in the nose that responds to pheromones (sex hormones) helps you know when you've found that special person. When you're with—or even think about—your beloved, your brain releases chemicals such as dopamine, a feel-good neurotransmitter, resulting in a pounding heart, dilated pupils, and flushed cheeks.

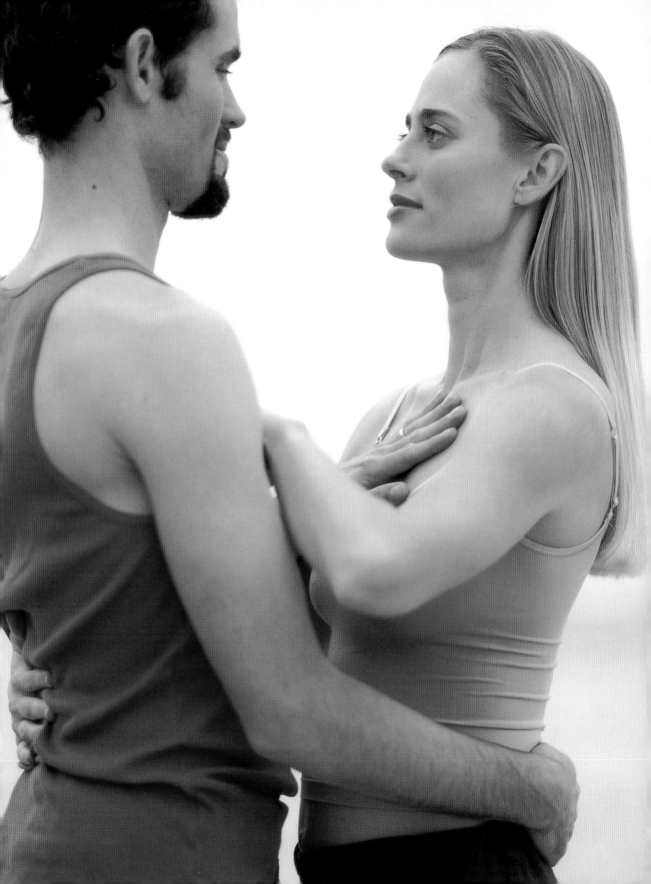

shampoo for two

Taking turns shampooing each other's hair creates a cascade of sensual pleasures, while promoting an intimacy with your partner based on touch and care.

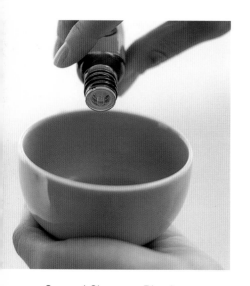

Sensual Shampoo Blend
6 to 8 ounces unscented shampoo
10 drops ylang-ylang essential oil
8 drops sandalwood essential oil
2 drops lavender essential oil

The combination of fragrant shampoo, a gentle head massage, and the splash of warm water on your hair and scalp is a treat most of us only get at a salon. But letting a loved one wash your hair—and then switching places—is a wonderful way to connect emotionally and indulge in truly caring for each other's wellbeing. Start by creating a shampoo infused with your favorite essential oils (see the recipe at left). Then choose a relaxing spot for the shampooing—it might be in the shower, the bathtub, or even outside in the garden.

To begin, pour warm water over your partner's hair. Rub a little shampoo between your hands. Working slowly from the front hairline toward the crown and from the side hairlines to the back, massage the shampoo into the scalp and hair in small, circular movements. Try to move the scalp with your fingertips, but don't dig in too hard (that hurts) or rub the hair too roughly (that damages hair shafts). Make the shampooing a leisurely process; this is as much about connecting with your partner as it is about cleaning his or her hair. Rinse the hair thoroughly with warm water and pat it dry with a towel.

WORKING UP A LATHER

A common misconception about shampoo is that its cleaning power is directly related to the amount of lather produced. Actually, some very fine, effective shampoos deliberately are formulated with reduced amounts of detergent, the component that causes the lather. Too much detergent strips hair of its natural oils, and since detergent is a pollutant, it isn't great for Mother Earth, either. Also remember to use a judicious amount of shampoo—unless your hair is very long or thick, a quarter-size dollop should do the job.

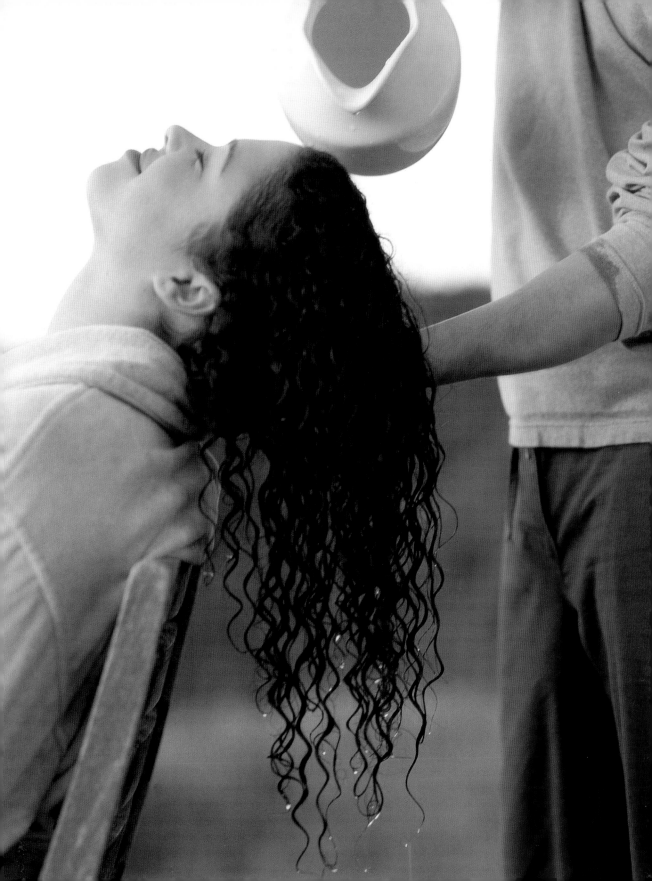

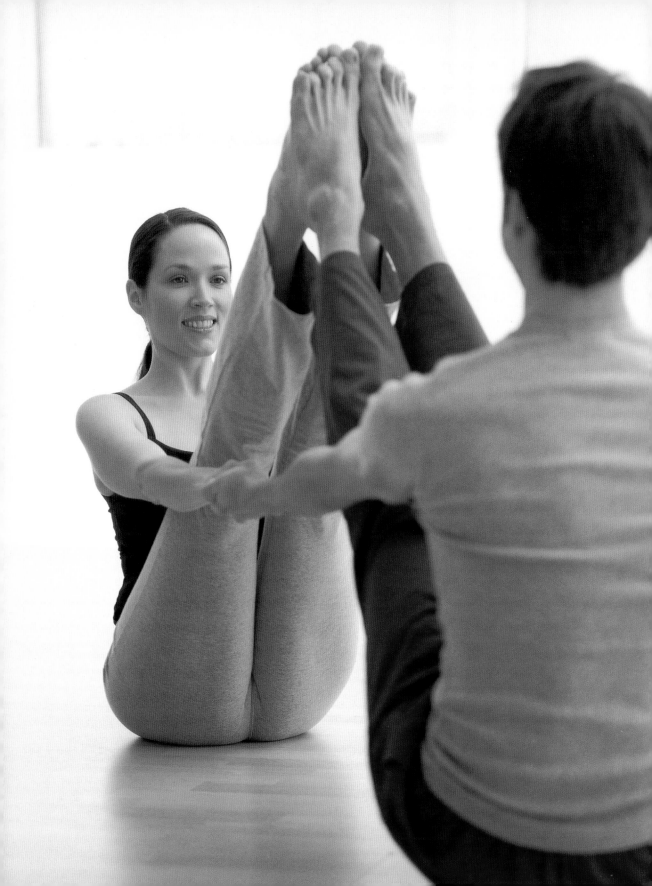

two boats

Feelings of connectedness, trust, and mutual support plus a glorious stretch—all are benefits of this intimate partner yoga pose that forms a striking silhouette.

This yoga pose is a double form of *Navasana*—the Boat—which earned its name for its supposed resemblance to a sailing ship. When done alone, the Boat pose is an extremely demanding pose, which requires strong abdominal muscles. Two Boats is a bit easier because you can use your partner to help brace your limbs and balance. A physical connection with your loved one also helps strengthen your emotional connection, as you depend upon each other for support and can enjoy the meditative aspects of yoga together.

To start, sit on the floor face-to-face with your partner. Bend your knees and put your feet flat on the floor, with the toes touching. Clasp each other's hands (or forearms, if that's more comfortable), then slowly lift and straighten your legs, one side at a time, letting the soles of your feet touch the soles of your partner's feet. Keep your back straight rather than rounding it. As you each balance on your buttocks, lift in and up from your lower back, gaze into each other's eyes, and breathe slowly and deeply. Hold this pose for at least 20 seconds, and, eventually, try to extend it to one minute.

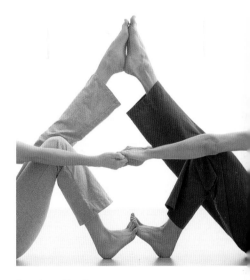

Steady as She Goes
The trick to getting into or out of the Two Boats yoga pose is to concentrate on one side at a time (do not try to lift both sets of legs simultaneously). As with any couple's pose, you must remain sensitive to each other's pace, position, and level of comfort.

GROWING CLOSER THROUGH YOGA

The Sanskrit word *yoga* means "union." Although usually applied to achieving harmony between one's own mind and body, the concept of yoga can also be applied to two individuals coming together as one. Poses such as Two Boats, Tree, and Double Dog allow a couple to share their passion for yoga—and one another. Even partners of dramatically different heights and weights can learn to balance and support each other, often under the watchful eye of an instructor at a couples-only yoga workshop.

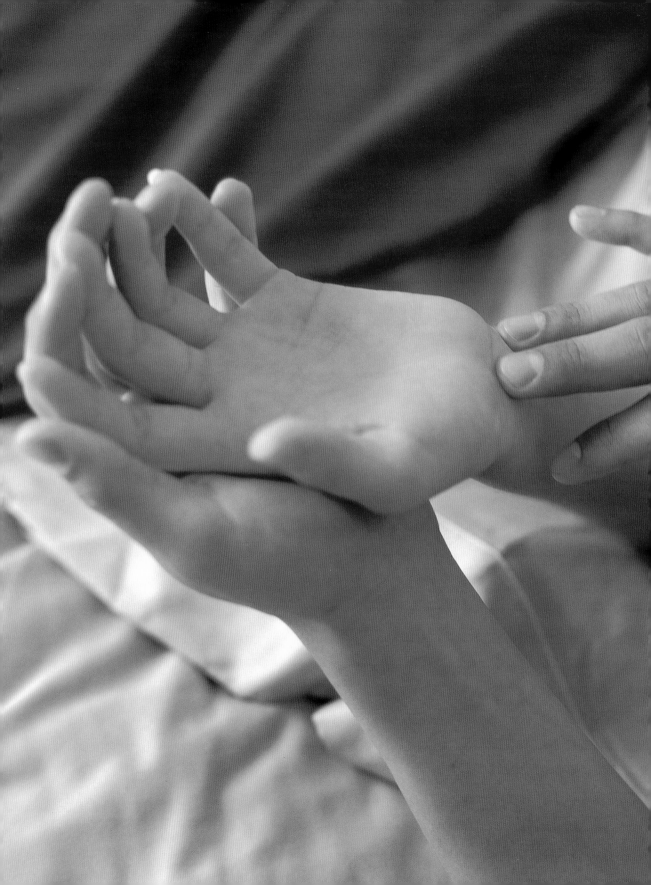

sensual massage

Get ready to turn up the heat with a loving massage.
The light strokes and attention to sensitive zones let
your partner explore you in an especially intimate way.

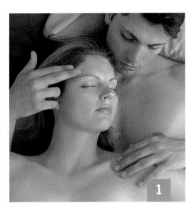

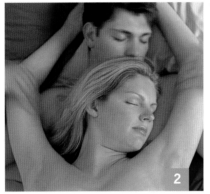

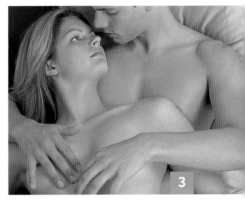

Begin this intimate massage with you and your partner resting
comfortably in bed. Lay your back against your partner's chest, and
ask him to follow these sensual massage steps:

1 Start by stroking along her forehead, between her eyebrows,
circling down along the cheekbones, and moving across to the bridge
of the nose. Slip your fingers down to your partner's lips; outline and
explore them with the gentlest touch. Then circle around her ears,
lightly tracing the outer rims and inner surfaces.

2 Continue your gentle caresses by stroking the soft, sensitive skin
of your partner's inner arms, elbows, and forearms. Then take your
partner's hand in yours and softly stroke the wrist and hand all the
way to the end of each fingertip. Repeat on the other hand.

3 Now move to the navel, and slowly trace your fingertips across
the belly and along the hips. Then trace inward along the waist to
the navel. Circle the navel a few times, and glide up the belly to the
breastbone. Continue to explore, lingering to circle sensitive spots.

Rubbing Your Partner the Right Way
As you massage your loved one,
experiment to find just the right
amount of pleasing pressure. You
want to use light, easy sweeps in
this sensual exercise, but if you
stroke too softly, you risk tickling,
not titillating, your partner.

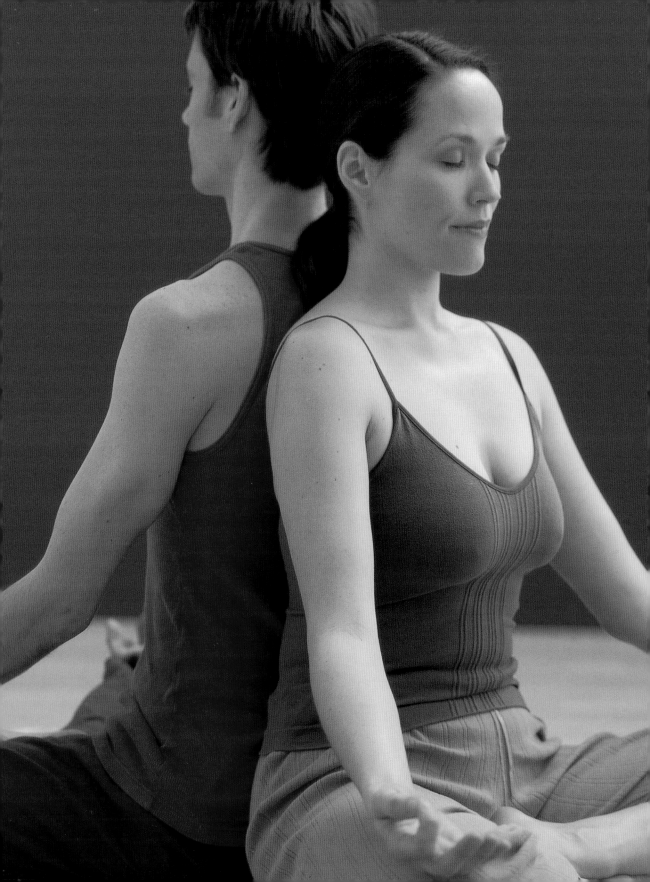

sharing breath

You share your thoughts, dreams, and embraces.
Now try sharing your breath with this yoga technique,
which can truly enhance your connectedness.

Sit on the floor or a bed in a meditative position with your back
resting against your partner's. The lights should be dim and the room
quiet. You also can listen to soft instrumental music or a recording
of nature sounds such as a gentle rainfall. Place your hands in a
comfortable position lightly on your knees or lap and close your
eyes; have your partner do the same. Focus on each other's breathing,
and begin to synchronize your slow, deep breaths. If you find your
mind wandering, bring it back to marking the regular pattern of your
inhalations and exhalations. Practice this for as long as you both like.

As a variation, give the Braided Rope pose a try. Sit cross-legged and
back-to-back with your partner as you inhale together and elongate
your spines. Then, placing your right hand on your left knee and
your left hand on the floor beside your left side (with your partner
doing the same), exhale as you each turn to your own left, keeping
your backs together as you twist. Hold for several breaths, then return
to center and repeat, this time rotating to your right. (See Hands to
Hearts on page 228 ◄ for another exercise in intimate contact.)

The Joy of Letting Go
By breathing slowly and deeply,
as you do in this yoga exercise,
you trigger your body's relaxation
response. Want proof? After taking
a half dozen deep breaths with your
partner, notice how your shoulders
naturally drop about a half inch or
so, signaling a release of tension.

SEX AND BREATHING

Although the shared breathing exercise described here is about
feeling peacefully connected (not all hot and bothered), breathing
also is at the root of many tantric sex practices. The tantric tradition
(which, despite what many Westerners think, is about much more
than sex) holds that deep, controlled breathing is a good way to
sharpen the senses and purify the body, readying it for the act of
love. When couples synchronize their breathing, it is seen as a
convergence of complementary masculine and feminine life forces.

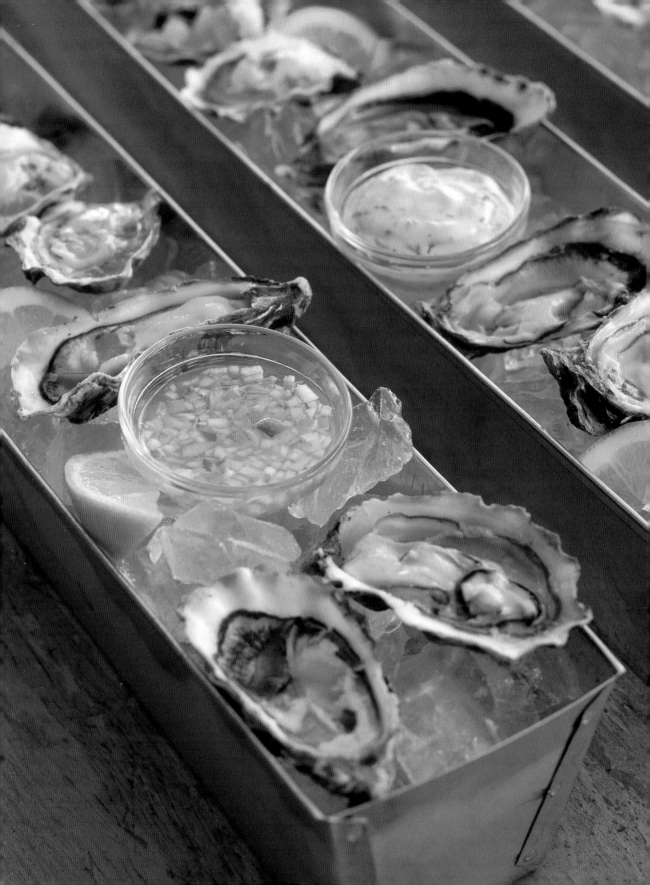

oysters for lovers

A plate of succulent fresh oysters accompanied by
a duo of luscious sauces just might help you set
the right mood for a romantic evening at home.

For purists, fresh oysters need very little to enhance their briny
beauty. But if it's variety you crave, a simple mignonette sauce strikes
a piquant note, while a crème fraîche sauce adds a touch of silken
sophistication. The key to success is to find extremely fresh oysters;
a reputable fishmonger is your best source and will open the oysters
and preserve the liquid for you. Thin slices of brown or pumpernickel
bread with butter is the classic accompaniment, as well as champagne.

1 To make the sherry mignonette sauce, combine the sherry wine
vinegar and shallot in a small bowl. Add the white pepper and one
drop of the jalapeño sauce. Adjust seasonings to taste and mix well.

2 To make the crème fraîche sauce, combine the crème fraîche,
mustard, dill, lemon zest and juice, and turmeric in a small bowl.
Add a pinch of salt and white pepper and mix well.

3 Line a platter with crushed ice. Arrange the oysters in their liquid
as well as the pair of sauces on the ice. Serve immediately.

Ingredients

3 tablespoons sherry wine vinegar

1 tablespoon minced shallot

Pinch of white pepper

1 drop Tabasco green jalapeño sauce

¼ cup crème fraîche

1 teaspoon Dijon mustard

1 to 2 teaspoons minced fresh dill

½ teaspoon lemon zest

1 teaspoon lemon juice

⅛ teaspoon turmeric

Pinch of Kosher salt and white pepper

1 dozen very fresh oysters

- Serves: 2
- Prep time: 10 minutes

FOOD TO PUT YOU IN THE MOOD

Truffles, chocolate, caviar, figs, honey, asparagus, shellfish, prunes,
camel's milk, sparrow brains, and skink flesh: All have reputations
as aphrodisiacs. But is there any scientific evidence that certain
foods can light up your libido? Alas, culinary aphrodisiacs remain
the stuff of folklore, according to the killjoys at Johns Hopkins
Medical Institutions; they report that "there is no scientific proof
that any food or beverage can increase desire." Taking the time to
prepare a special meal, however, remains a lovely way to express
affection. Best to skip the sparrow brains and skink flesh, however.

Nutritional Information Per Serving
The following data is for a half dozen
oysters and both dipping sauces.

Calories	179
Kilojoules	750
Protein	7 g
Carbohydrates	6 g
Total Fat	13 g
Saturated Fat	7 g
Cholesterol	72 mg
Sodium	180 mg
Dietary Fiber	0 g

relax

We live in an age when going 24/7 is viewed as a laudable goal, not a warning sign. To restore balance and a sense of sanity, step out of the fray and practice the fine art of relaxation.

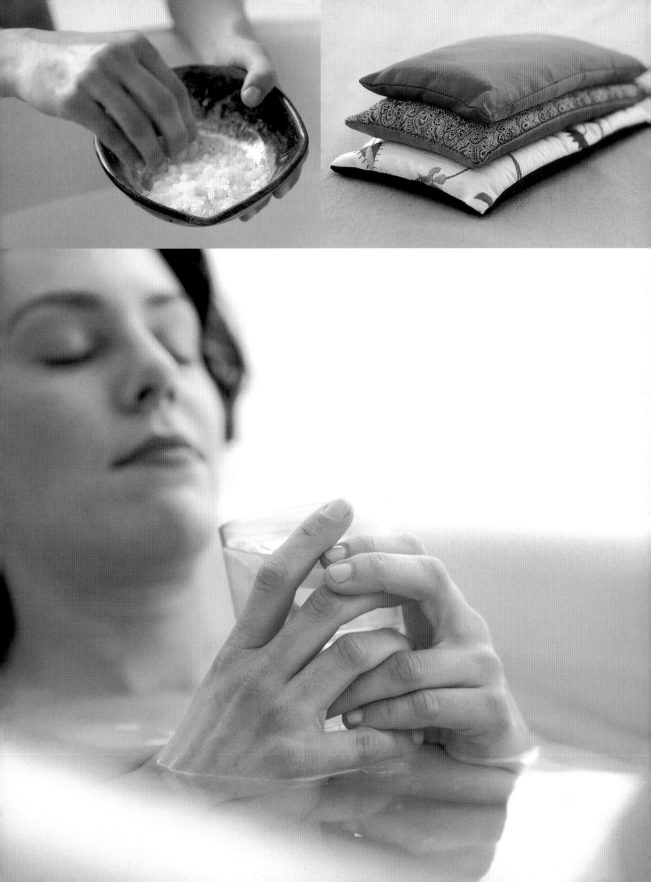

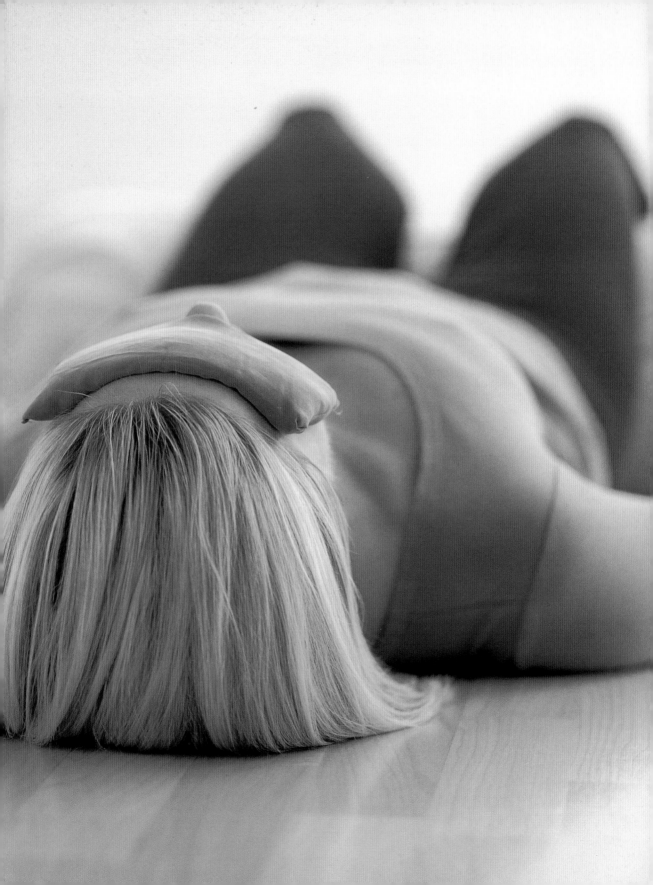

relax

Just as muscles need time to recover between strength-training sessions, your entire being needs time to unclench between periods of intense effort and the whirlwind of activities that no doubt mark your days. As the saying goes, all work and no play makes for a dull girl. Not to mention a frazzled, exhausted, and cranky one.

Taking the time to daydream, stretch, and observe the world around you can yield some amazing dividends. Your mind clears, your body recovers, and your spirit soars. On the following pages, you'll find a variety of avenues to help you discover your own personal path to true relaxation. You might swap back massages with your partner or a friend. You might be lulled by the satisfying stirring of a gently bubbling risotto. Perhaps you'll opt for the energy boost that comes from a tai chi session or the release provided by yogic breathing.

Just remember that letting things go can be as important as getting them done. In fact, letting go is sometimes the best way to ensure you do your best. After all, a relaxed body moves more freely. A calm mind hears its muse more easily. And a tranquil heart can better feel the emotions that make us human, including love and joy.

relax

gathering chi

Tai chi practitioners believe that you can increase the amount of *chi*, life's vital energy, in your body by gathering it from the air and the universe.

1 Stand tall, with tailbone tucked in, knees gently bent, chin slightly down, feet shoulder-width apart, and arms hanging down, relaxed.

2 As you slowly squat, bring your arms out to create a large circle, as if you're about to pick up a beach ball. Make sure your elbows, wrists, and knees stay relaxed, your arms are rounded and wide, and your hands never quite touch each other as you gather up the ball.

3 Stand up again, and as you rise, bring your arms in toward your abdomen, as if you were trying to push the air out of the ball.

4 Now look up and raise your arms, keeping them rounded, as if reaching for another ball. Then bring your arms in toward your waist again, as if trying to deflate the ball. Drop your hands to your sides, and repeat the steps for three to five minutes.

The Sources of Chi

In Eastern traditions, chi comes from a variety of sources. We each inherit a certain amount from our parents (this kind of chi is called *jing*). Other chi comes from the food we eat (with wholesome food possessing more chi than unhealthy food) and the air we breathe (the less polluted the better). Finally, some of our chi is derived from the universe itself.

THE SEVEN CHAKRAS

In tai chi, yoga, and Eastern medicine, the body's *prana* (life force) is believed to flow along energy channels that intersect at *chakras* (or wheels), which are associated with distinct states of mind.

CHAKRA	LOCATION	ASSOCIATED WITH
First	Base of spine	Security, wellbeing
Second	Just beneath navel	Sensuality, fertility
Third	Solar plexus	Personal power, belonging
Fourth	Heart	Love, generosity
Fifth	Throat	Creativity, communication
Sixth	Between eyebrows	Intuition, awareness
Seventh	Top of head	Spirituality

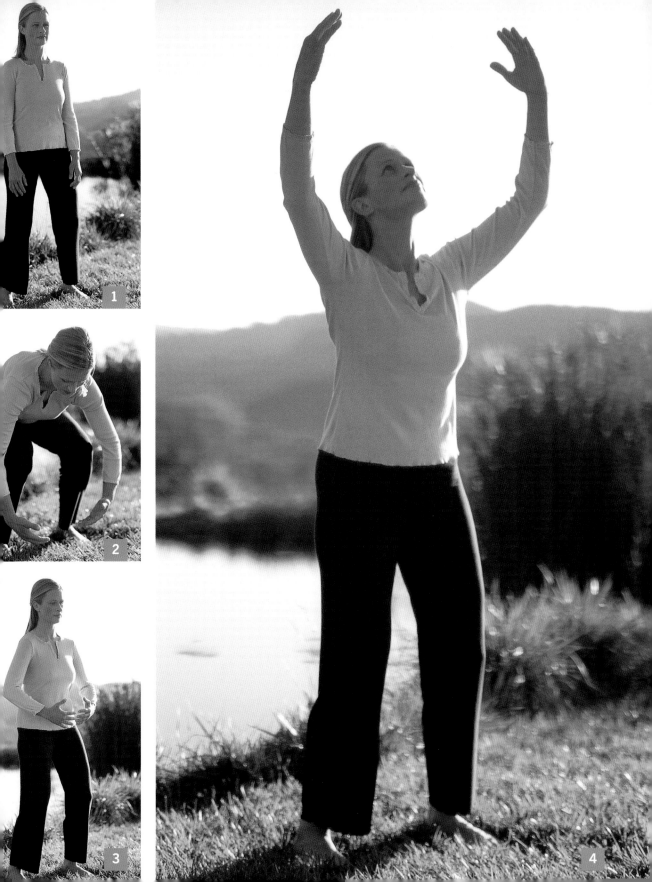

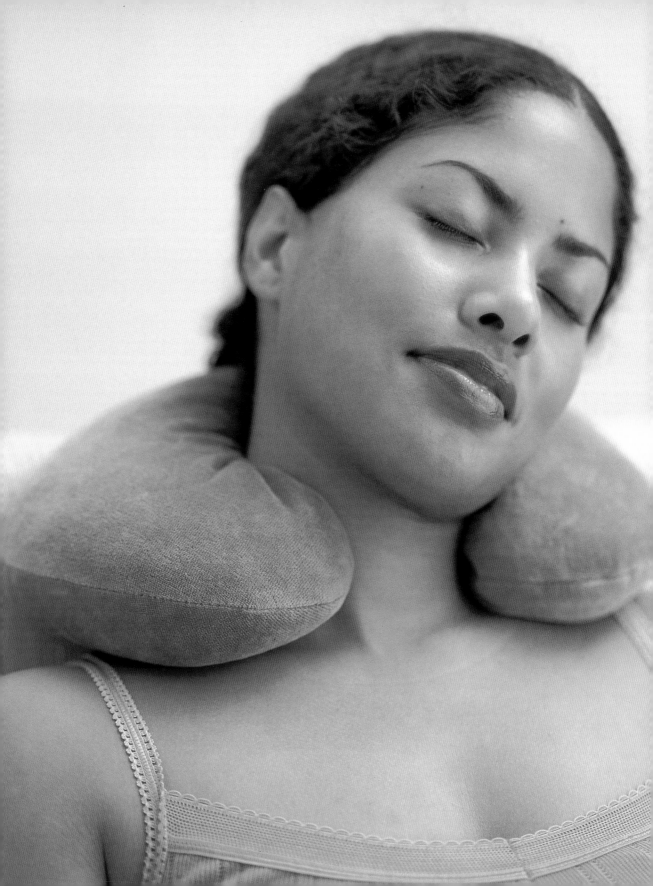

soothing neck wrap

After a hard day of working, running errands, or taking care of the kids, give yourself a treat and provide your aching muscles with a scented, heated neck wrap.

Need to be convinced of the stress that builds up in your neck and shoulders every day? Just try doing a few side-to-side head rolls or a couple of shoulder shrugs to feel those kinks, aching muscles, and sore spots come alive. But help is at hand: Using a specially designed neck wrap or pillow can ease some of the tension and discomfort and allow for a much greater range of movement with your neck.

Purchase a heatable wrap or soft pillow that conforms well to the contours of your neck and is filled with rice and aromatic herbs. The weight of the rice puts subtle pressure on your muscles, helping to loosen them; the scent of the herbs is calming to frazzled nerves; and the heat helps melt away tension and soreness.

To enhance the relaxing effect of this treatment, you might want to sprinkle a few drops of essential oil onto your neck wrap or pillow. Pick a soothing scent that goes well with any herbs or other plants already contained in the wrap. For example, jasmine harmonizes with lavender, and chamomile complements rosemary. Bergamot is an especially soothing and reassuring scent that blends well with many other aromatic oils, including cypress, ginger, palmarosa, juniper, lemon, neroli, ylang-ylang, or geranium. If you're using a pure essential oil, be sure to mix it with a little carrier oil before sprinkling it on the pillow to avoid skin irritation.

Find a quiet spot to sit where you can lean back with your head supported, such as an upholstered, high-back chair. Heat the pillow or wrap as directed by its manufacturer, and place it behind your neck, on top of your shoulders. Sit back and relax for about ten minutes, or until the pillow or wrap cools and your tension has faded away—at least until you face tomorrow's challenges.

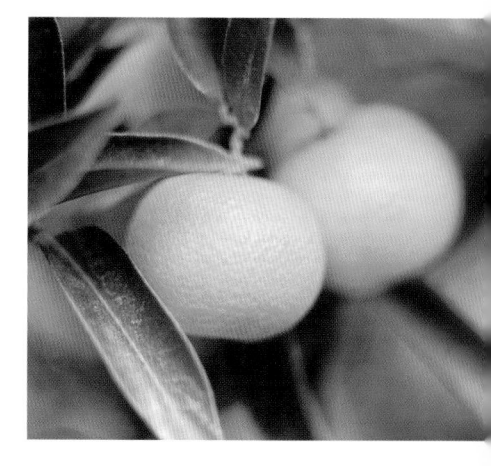

The Beauty of Bergamot
Bergamot's bright, citrusy flavor gives Earl Grey tea its distinctive taste. Its essential oil, which is distilled from the peel of the fruit, has been used for medicinal and skin-care purposes since Renaissance times. Bergamot's scent is considered extremely uplifting and soothing; aromatherapists recommend it for treating anxiety, anger, fear, and even mild depression.

mountain poses

Yoga poses that involve balancing help you better understand the interplay between movement and stillness. They also can improve your posture.

Blind Ambition

If you'd like to make any standing yoga poses more challenging, try doing them with your eyes closed. It's trickier than you might think to maintain your balance when you lose your point of visual reference.

Start with the basic Mountain yoga pose (see the photo at right): Stand with your feet together and your arms relaxed at your sides to form a long, straight line with your body. Tighten your quadriceps (the muscles on the front of your thighs) to help stabilize your knees and prevent them from locking. Keep your chin up and head facing forward. Release your shoulder blades so they are down and loose, keeping your collarbones lifted and wide. Relax the muscles of your face and throat. Challenge your balancing skills by closing your eyes. Hold for several breaths, visualizing the steadiness of a mountain.

Praying Mountain is a variation on this pose. Stand, as before, tall and straight with your feet together. Instead of resting your arms by your sides, hold your hands in the prayer position (palms pressed together, fingers pointing up) and bring them up to chest level. Distribute your weight evenly on both feet, tighten your quadriceps, keep your shoulders dropped, and stand tall. Hold for several breaths.

TRIANGLE OF STABILITY

To help maintain your balance when performing the Mountain and similar poses, fix your gaze on a point at or just below eye level in front of you. Visualize a triangle of stability being created between your eyes, your chosen point of focus, and your center of gravity (just below your navel). Learning to balance this way will help you achieve a new level of equilibrium and experience the freedom of physical and mental poise. Don't push yourself too hard on this notion, though. If you're having trouble balancing, practice these poses near or against a wall. As your body and mind strengthen, you'll be able to give up the external support.

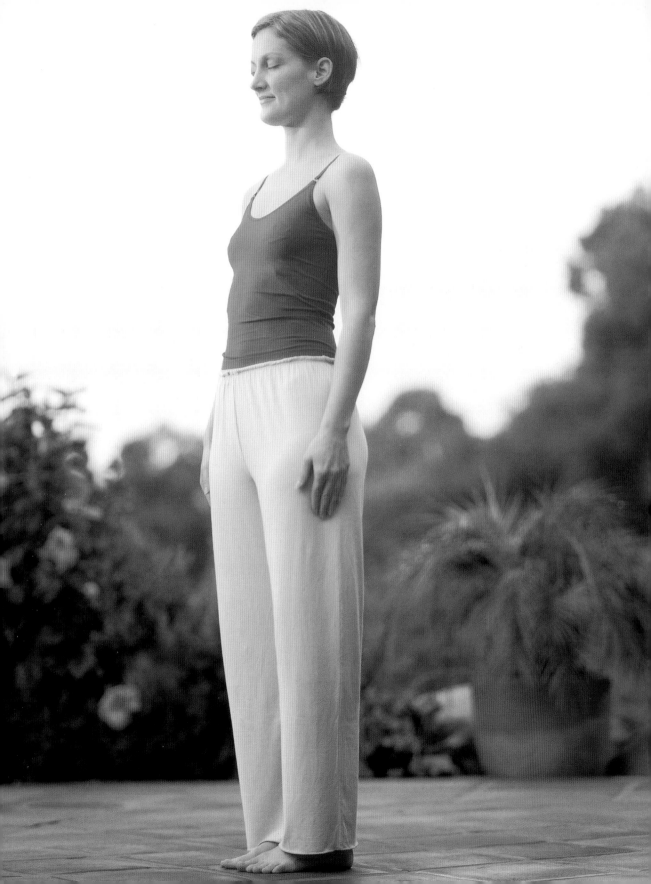

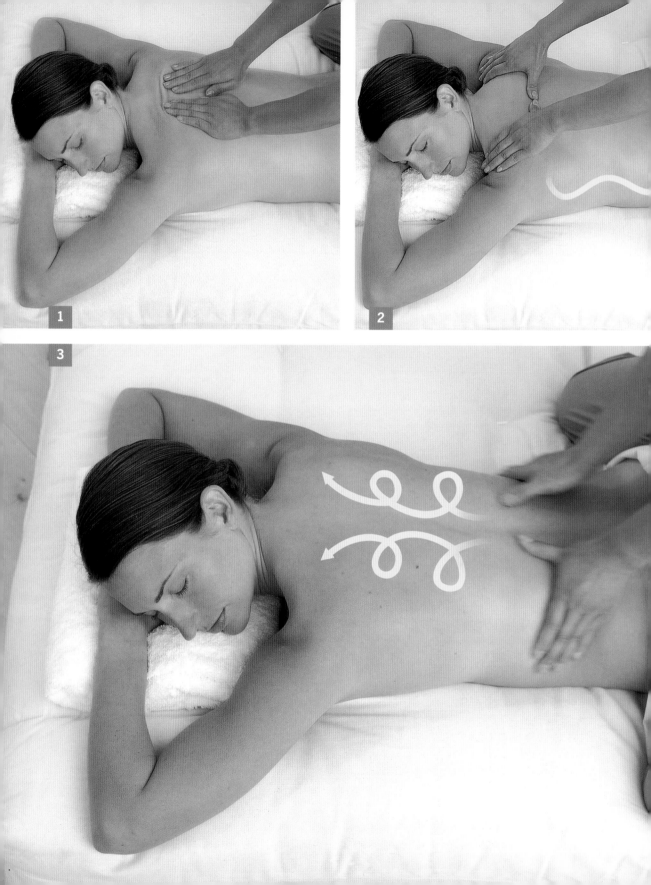

1

2

3

back-friendly massage

Whether coping with aches and pains or just aiming for a little overall relaxation, these techniques help relax the often tense and sore muscles of the back.

Ask a friend to follow these simple massage steps:

1 After warming some massage oil in your hands (see the recipe at right), glide up the thick muscles alongside the spine. Press firmly with your fingertips and palms, and contour your hands to fit the shape of her back as you glide. At the base of the neck, fan out your hands and stroke across the top and down the sides of her shoulders.

2 Curve your hands around the shoulders and pull down toward the ribs. Glide down the sides toward the hips, sweep your fingers under the waist, then lean back and gently pull toward you to stretch out the muscles of the lower back. Repeat Steps 1 and 2 four more times.

3 Starting on the lower back, press your thumbs into the muscles on each side of the spine. Using firm pressure, circle your thumbs into the muscles as you gradually make your way up to the neck. Always be careful to press to the side of, never directly on, the spine. Then circle your thumbs into the muscles around the base of the neck and across her shoulders. Repeat three more times.

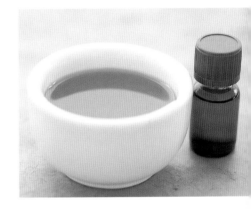

Back-to-Basics Massage Blend

2 ounces carrier oil (such as sweet
    almond, grape seed, or jojoba)

12 drops lavender essential oil

8 drops clary sage essential oil

5 drops ylang-ylang essential oil

BACK PAIN IN WOMEN

Men and women often differ in the kinds and causes of back pain they endure. A woman's back pain typically lasts longer than a man's and tends to constrain her activities more; men, though, have a higher risk of recurrence. A man's pain often results from a sudden injury, but a woman's usually stems from the cumulative strain of routine activities, such as gardening. Pregnant women often suffer back pain because they deal with a shifted center of balance by throwing back their shoulders and overarching the lumbar area.

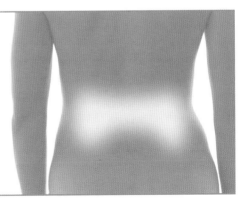

taking the waters

Even if you can't get away to a luxurious spa, you can enjoy some of the benefits of a spa at home by preparing your own restorative mineral bath.

For centuries, Europeans have delighted in "taking the waters," soaking in and imbibing mineral water from hot springs known for their curative and restorative powers. At celebrated spas from Bath to Budapest, hydrotherapy treatments are used to treat a host of ailments, including neurological illnesses, gastrointestinal disorders, arthritis, gynecological problems, and respiratory difficulties. Many spa clients also believe that hydrotherapy is the closest thing they'll ever find to the fountain of youth, crediting the waters with the power to keep them looking and feeling young. We can't promise the mineral-water treatment described here will provide such wondrous results, but it will go a long way toward enhancing your sense of general wellbeing and making you feel wonderfully relaxed.

First, pour yourself a tall glass of chilled mineral water and place it within easy reach of your bathtub. If you like, you can add a slice of lime, lemon, or cucumber to make it even more refreshing. Then fill your bathtub with very warm water, enough to completely cover your shoulders. Add a handful of scented mineral bath salts to the water and mix them with your hand until they completely dissolve. Ease into the tub, lie back (use a bath pillow or rolled-up towel to cradle your neck, if you like), and close your eyes. Rest in your hot, softening bath for at least 20 minutes, breathing slowly and deeply.

Since you're immersing yourself in very warm water, you'll perspire, so it's important to keep your body well hydrated. Sip from your glass of cool mineral water frequently as you soak. After you've finished bathing and have dried yourself off, be sure to refill your water glass and keep it nearby; you'll want to continue drinking plenty of water after the treatment to help flush out any released toxins.

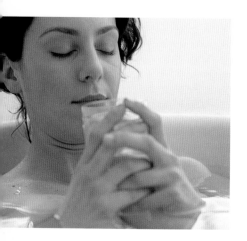

Fresh from the Source
To earn the official designation "mineral water," the water must originate from an underground source, be collected directly from where it emerged from the ground, contain a certain amount of naturally occurring minerals and other trace elements, and be free of pollution.

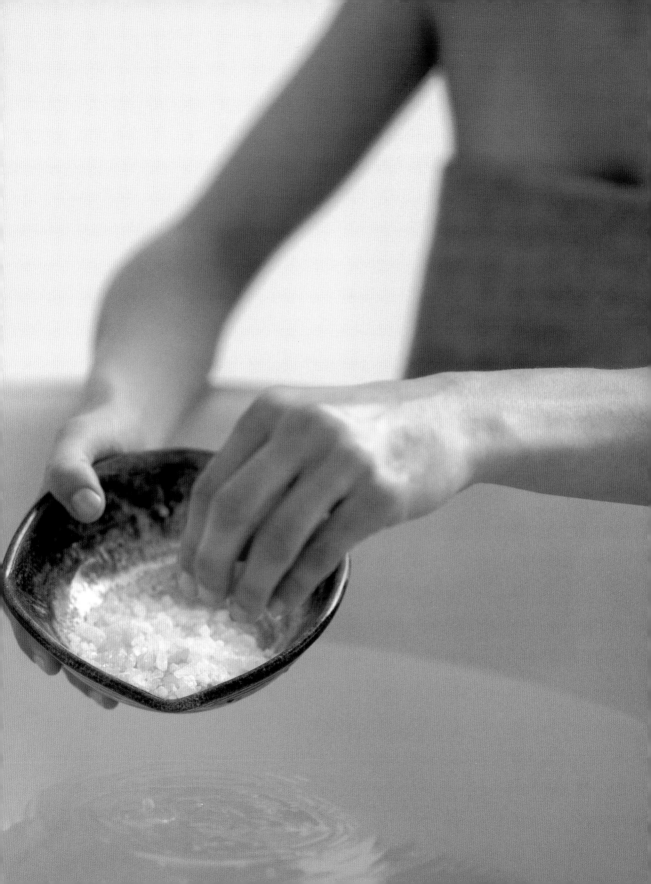

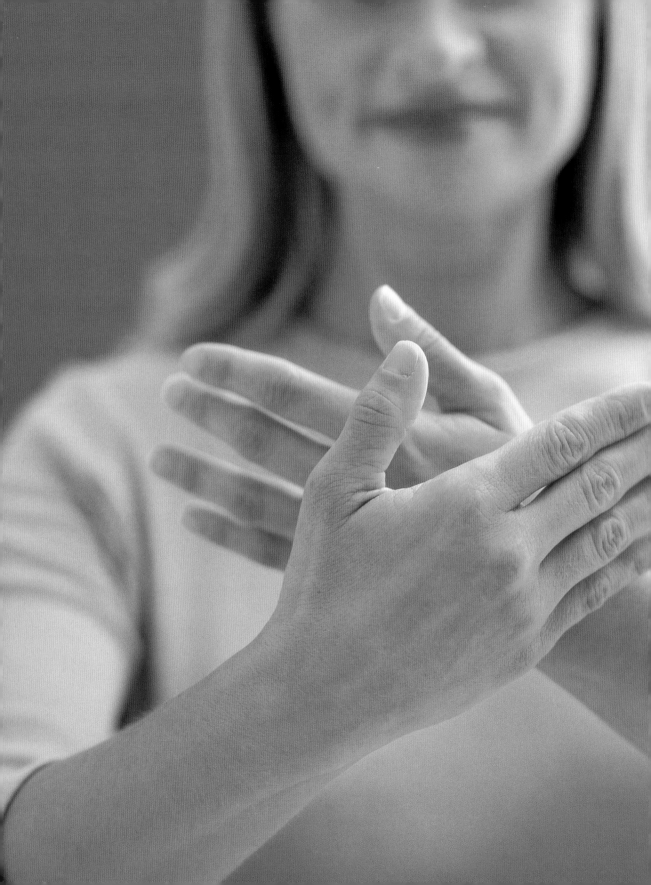

tai chi closing sequence

Feeling wound up? This calming, soothing, and meditative tai chi sequence will help you unwind, whether you do it after an exercise session or simply a long day of work.

We all know the feeling of having too much pent-up energy in our bodies—that anxious sense of having been overstimulated, overcaffeinated, or just generally overwrought by the course of daily events. That shouldn't happen during a tai chi session, but tai chi practitioners still believe it's important to settle down the body's *chi* (or energy) after completing a form (or series of tai chi movements). That's because this ancient internal and martial art focuses on both gathering and stimulating the flow of chi; if that energy isn't calmed, it can leave the practitioner feeling scattered or not centered. (For more information about chi, see page 244 ◄.)

The flowing arm movements in the following tai chi exercise are believed to help push the chi down and settle it. If you're having trouble picturing this, think of smoothing out wrinkled sheets or a slightly mussed tablecloth. Some tai chi practitioners also compare these movements to those of the setting sun. However you envision them, remember this: The overriding goal is to preserve the energy in the body, yet to relax it in a calm, meditative fashion.

HOW LONG DOES IT TAKE TO SEE RESULTS?

You'll probably feel more relaxed and graceful after your first couple of weeks of tai chi sessions, but keep it up for a few months and you'll likely experience even greater results. One U.S. study found that elderly women's scores on balance and mobility increased "significantly" after they practiced tai chi for three months. Another study conducted in the U.S. found that after six months of tai chi classes, older adults felt more confident physically and also had more strength, a greater range of motion, and better balance.

step-by-step sequence ►

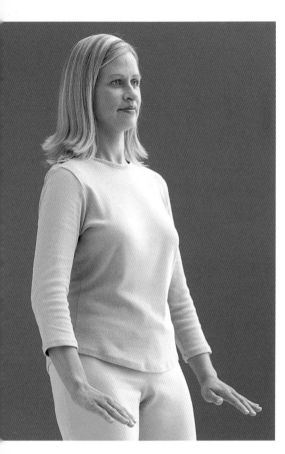

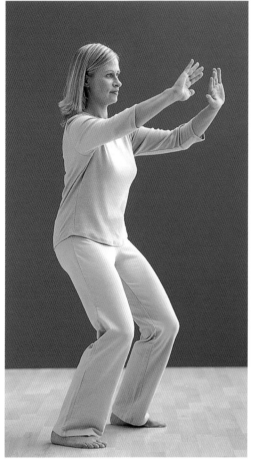

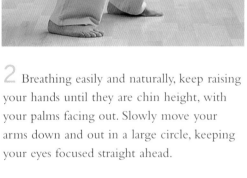

1 Stand with your feet shoulder-width apart and toes pointing straight ahead. Start with your arms relaxed by your sides. Go into a shallow squat, keeping your tailbone tucked in, eyes straight ahead, and knees relaxed. As you sink down, start to raise your hands.

2 Breathing easily and naturally, keep raising your hands until they are chin height, with your palms facing out. Slowly move your arms down and out in a large circle, keeping your eyes focused straight ahead.

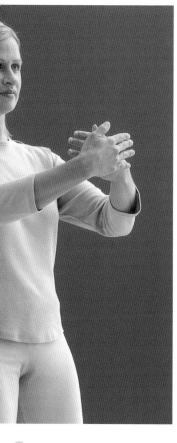
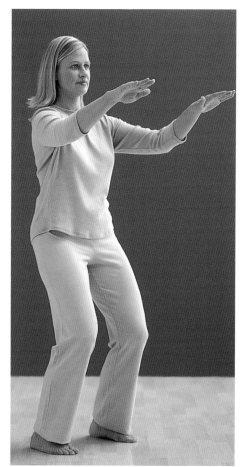
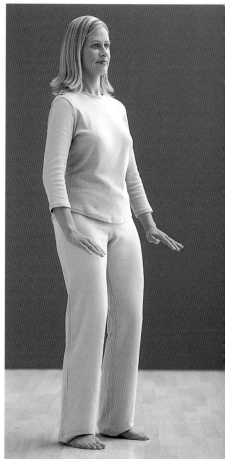

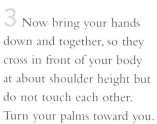 3 Now bring your hands down and together, so they cross in front of your body at about shoulder height but do not touch each other. Turn your palms toward you.

4 Turn your palms to face the ground and begin to stretch your hands out in front of you, as if you were pushing them along the surface of a table. Your shoulders should be dropped and relaxed.

5 Keeping your feet hip-width apart, rise out of the squat, and let your arms sink down and rest by your sides. End by taking a step in with one foot. Repeat Steps 1 through 5 four times.

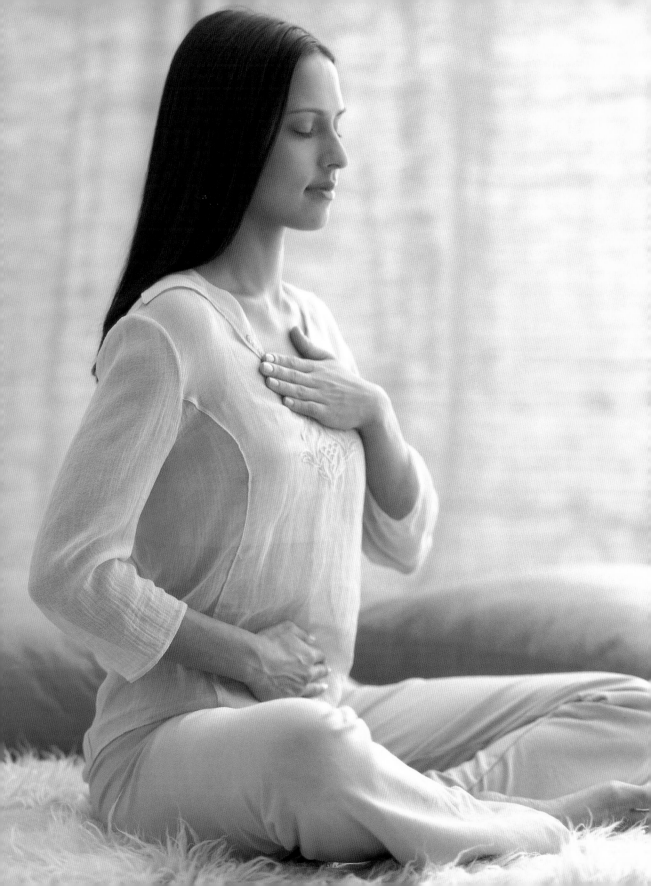

full yogic breath

By bringing you into the moment and expanding the capacity of your lungs, this traditional yoga breathing practice provides a ticket to profound relaxation.

Called *Deergha Swaasam* in Sanskrit, the Full Yogic Breath has long been thought to help practitioners develop concentration, clarity, and attunement with the heavens because it allows them to conjure up so much *prana,* or life force. It also is extremely relaxing.

To begin the breathing exercise, sit comfortably on the floor or in a chair. Inhale through your nostrils from your abdomen upward, expanding your belly and rib cage, then lifting your collarbones with the rise of your breath. Try to use the full capacity of your lungs. Then exhale in the opposite order: first letting the area just below the collarbones empty of breath, then your rib cage, and finally your abdomen. If it's hard for you to track the course of your breath (this becomes easier with practice), put one hand on your abdomen and the other on your chest, so you can feel your body moving with your inhalations and exhalations. Just breathe slowly and deeply this way for a few minutes as you enjoy this calm, contemplative state.

Every Breath You Take
Most people breathe about 12 times per minute—or approximately 17,000 breaths per day—to fill the body's daily need for 88 pounds of oxygen. Most of that breathing goes unnoticed, unless we begin breathing harder to get more oxygen to our muscles—for example, when we're exercising. In those instances, we can breathe 60 times or more per minute.

THE BENEFITS OF DEEP BREATHING
You hear it all the time: "Relax and take a deep breath." Although those who proffer this common piece of advice may not realize it, the notion actually is based on a bodily process known as the Hering-Breuer reflex. When you inhale fully and slowly, receptors in your lungs signal your cardiovascular system to relax, triggering a decrease in heart rate. In addition, deep breathing floods your body with oxygen—its primary fuel—and opens your chest, which yogis say stimulates the heart chakra (see page 244 ◄), a chakra associated with love and expansiveness. Simply breathing deeply and slowly can calm and nourish you anytime, anyplace.

neck rubs

Recruit a friend to give you a stress-busting neck massage that will undo all those knots and kinks and help get your mind thinking clearly again.

Massage for the Masses
If you lack the time or money for a full-blown massage, you can reap some of the same benefits by indulging in one of the quick and economical "chair massages" that seem to be popping up everywhere. Usually about 15 minutes in length, these rubdowns involve sitting in a specially designed chair with all your clothes on while the masseuse or masseur (generally a certified massage therapist) goes to work on your neck, shoulders, and upper back. Chair massages are available in all sorts of convenient places these days, including airports, sports events, malls, car dealerships, corporate offices, convention centers —even grocery stores.

To prepare for this relaxing massage treatment, sit backward astride a comfortable chair and rest both of your palms on the back of the chair. Then have your friend follow these step-by-step directions:

1 Standing behind the chair, lean your forearms on top of your friend's shoulders and press down with one arm. Hold for three slow breaths, then release. Repeat with the other arm. Then press down with both forearms simultaneously as your friend inhales and lifts her shoulders, pushing them into your forearms. On the exhale, keep pressing as your friend relaxes and rolls her head in a slow circle.

2 Have your friend rest her forehead in her hands and place her elbows on the back of the chair. Now press with the pad of one of your thumbs into the muscles at the base of the skull. You should use firm pressure, but check to make sure she isn't feeling any discomfort. Sink your thumb in on the inhale, and release on the exhale. Work point by point upward and outward along one side of the neck to about an inch behind her ear. Repeat this step on the other side.

3 With slightly cupped hands, press the pads of your fingers into the muscles on both sides of the spine, near the base of her skull. Using small circling motions, travel down to the base of the neck. Repeat this technique three more times.

4 Then hold her forehead with one hand. Grip the back of her neck with the thumb and fingers of your other hand and gently rub back and forth across the neck muscles on each side of the spine, working from an inch below the earlobes down to the base of the neck. Slowly increase your pressure as you feel the muscles start to loosen. Do three sets of these massage moves.

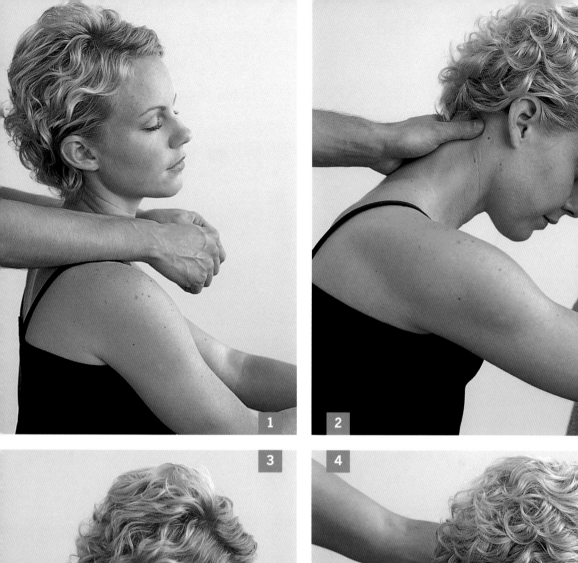

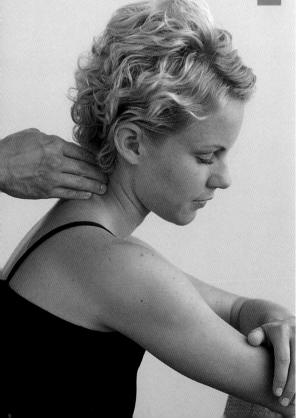

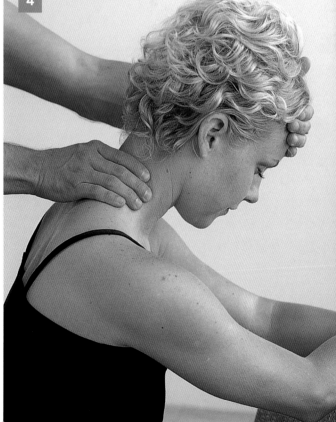

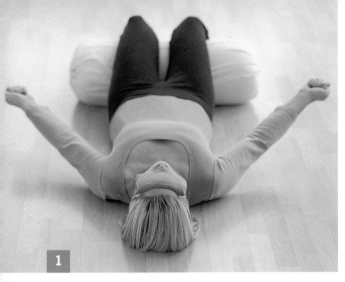

1

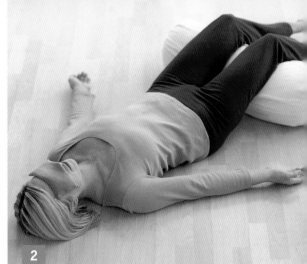

2

3

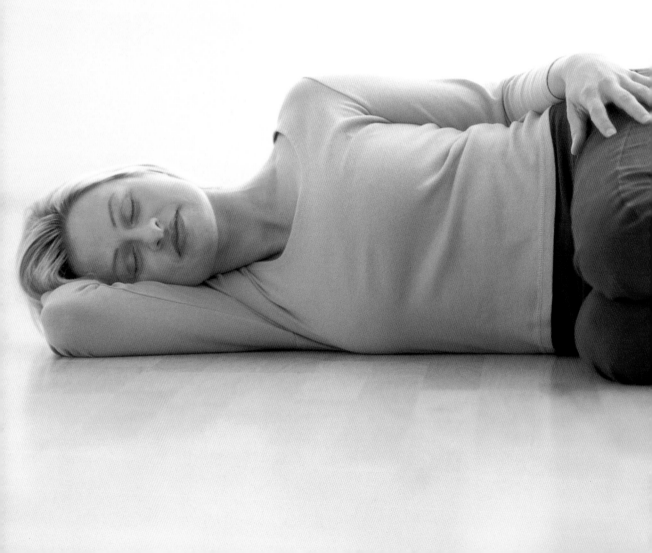

post-yoga bliss

Deep relaxation is a form of meditation that traditionally is performed at the end of a yoga session to allow the benefits of the poses to thoroughly permeate your body.

1 Lie on your back. For additional comfort, you might want to lie on a carpeted floor or yoga mat with a pillow underneath your knees and a soothing eye pillow over your eyes. Inhale and, holding your breath, make fists as you lift your arms several inches from the floor. Squeeze your fists for a few seconds; exhale and relax, letting your arms drop to the floor. Now inhale, and then hold your breath as you lift your legs and contract your leg muscles. Exhale and let your legs drop. Next, inhale deeply to puff out your belly; release as you exhale. Repeat with your chest. Then gently rock your head from side to side for a few seconds. Scrunch up your face; then relax it.

2 Mentally scan your body, spending a few moments on each part as you gradually shift your focus from your toes to the top of your head. If you sense any tension as you scan, visualize that particular area softening and relaxing. You might imagine a wave of warm light slowly rising through your body, creating a perfect state of physical ease. Now observe the natural ebb and flow of your breath. After about a minute, notice the thoughts that arise in your mind, but try not to have any feelings attached to them. After another minute, take the awareness even deeper, to your inner center of blissful calm. Allow yourself to fully experience this bliss for several minutes.

3 As you prepare to rouse yourself from this state of deep relaxation, spend a minute deepening your breath and enjoying the focused calm you have evoked. Then roll slowly over to your right side, cradling your right arm beneath your head; bend your knees and bring them toward your chest. When you feel ready to sit up, rise slowly. Although you are reentering the everyday world, this feeling of blissful calm will linger, leaving you refreshed and renewed.

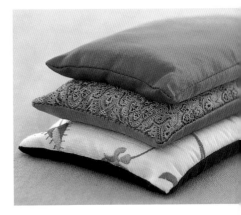

The Soothing Effect of Eye Pillows
An eye pillow can add another dimension to your meditation. Made of soft fabric such as cotton or silk, and filled with ingredients such as buckwheat hulls and flaxseed, these pillows block out light and soothe overworked eyes by pressing upon them gently. Some can be cooled or heated, while others contain calming aromatic herbs such as chamomile or lavender.

relax

risotto primavera

The very act of making risotto is relaxing—all that satisfying stirring of the rice as it plumps up so nicely. And your reward? A bowl of supremely comforting food.

Ingredients

1 pound fava bean pods
8 asparagus spears (1-inch pieces)
4 to 5 cups vegetable or chicken broth
¼ cup extra-virgin olive oil
½ cup thinly sliced green onions
1½ cups Arborio rice
1 garlic clove, minced
⅓ cup dry white wine
½ cup finely diced zucchini
½ cup grated Parmesan cheese
Kosher salt and freshly ground pepper
¼ cup chopped fresh Italian parsley
½ cup chopped fresh basil leaves

- Serves: 4
- Prep time: 25 minutes
- Cooking time: 25 minutes

Nutritional Information Per Serving

Fava beans (or broad beans) are low in fat and rich in fiber and protein.

Calories	380
Kilojoules	1,580
Protein	15 g
Carbohydrates	57 g
Total Fat	11 g
Saturated Fat	3 g
Cholesterol	10 mg
Sodium	900 mg
Dietary Fiber	7 g

Risotto accented with slender asparagus spears, fava beans, zucchini, and fresh herbs brings spring to the table. It's one dish that can't be rushed; the very process of making risotto forces you to slow down and lets you savor the fresh ingredients as you wash and chop the vegetables and then coax the pearly rice to absorb the broth.

1 Remove the fava beans from their pods (they should yield about ½ cup of shelled beans). Blanch the beans in boiling water for one minute and drain. When cooled, remove the skin of each bean.

2 Blanch the asparagus pieces for one minute. Drain and set the asparagus aside. Reserve the tips for garnish.

3 Heat the chicken or vegetable broth in a medium saucepan. Keep it at a gentle simmer throughout the cooking process.

4 In a large saucepan, warm the olive oil over medium heat. Add the onion, and sauté two to three minutes until the onion has softened. Add the rice and minced garlic, and stir for three to four minutes, until the grains start to turn translucent.

5 Add the wine, and continue to stir. When the liquid is almost completely absorbed by the rice, add about ½ cup of the hot broth. Stir frequently, adding ½ cup of hot broth at a time as the liquid gets absorbed. Do not let the rice dry out! After about 12 minutes, add the zucchini, fava beans, and asparagus. Continue adding broth and stirring until the rice is firm but tender—another six minutes or so.

6 Remove the saucepan from the heat. Stir in the Parmesan cheese. Add salt and pepper to taste. Stir in the parsley and basil. Place in a large warmed bowl and garnish with the reserved asparagus tips. Serve extra Parmesan to be sprinkled on the risotto at the table.

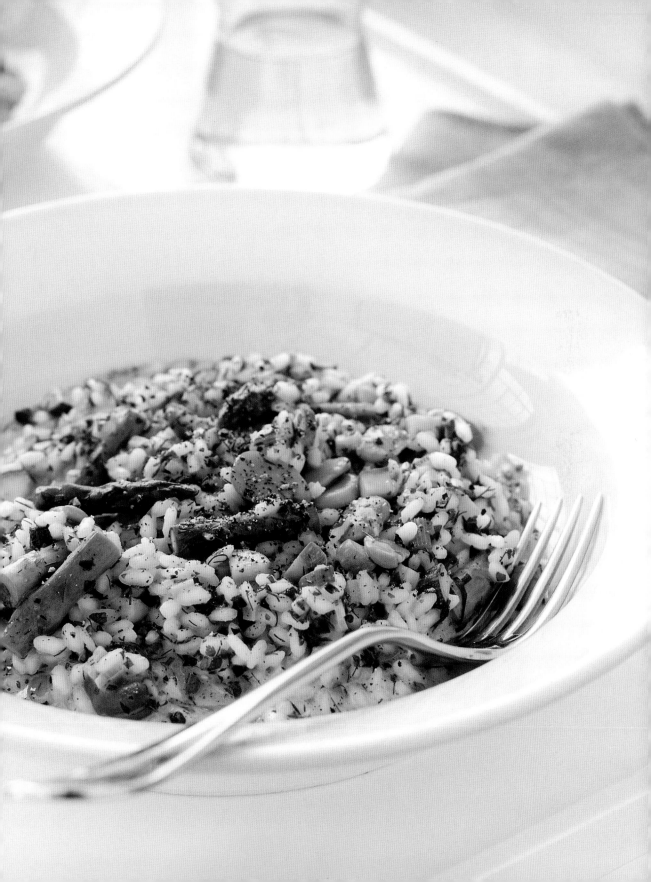

indulge

Too often, the term "indulgence" is linked to guilty pleasures. But it can also involve healthy and uplifting practices that let you partake in a little of the self-care you richly deserve.

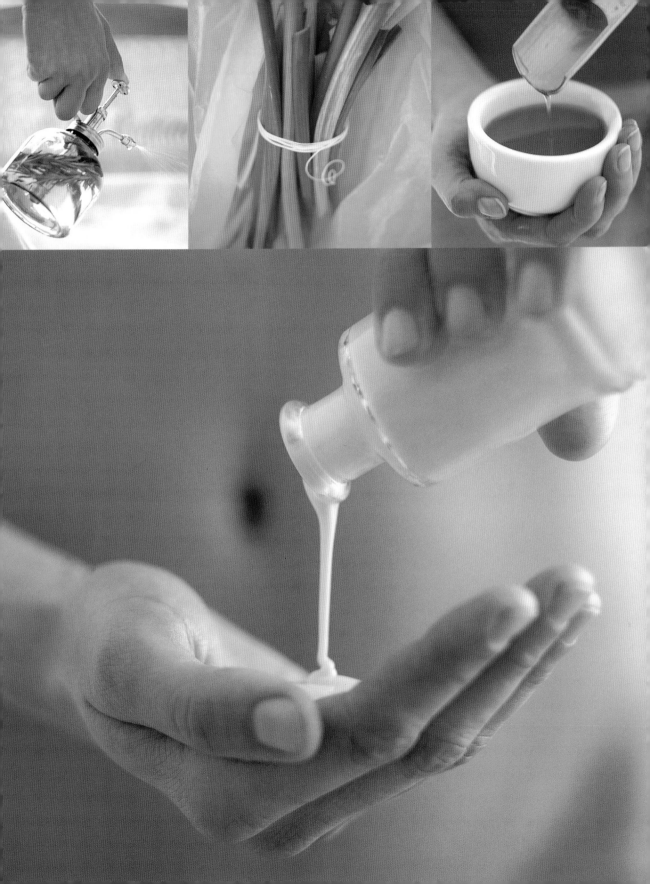

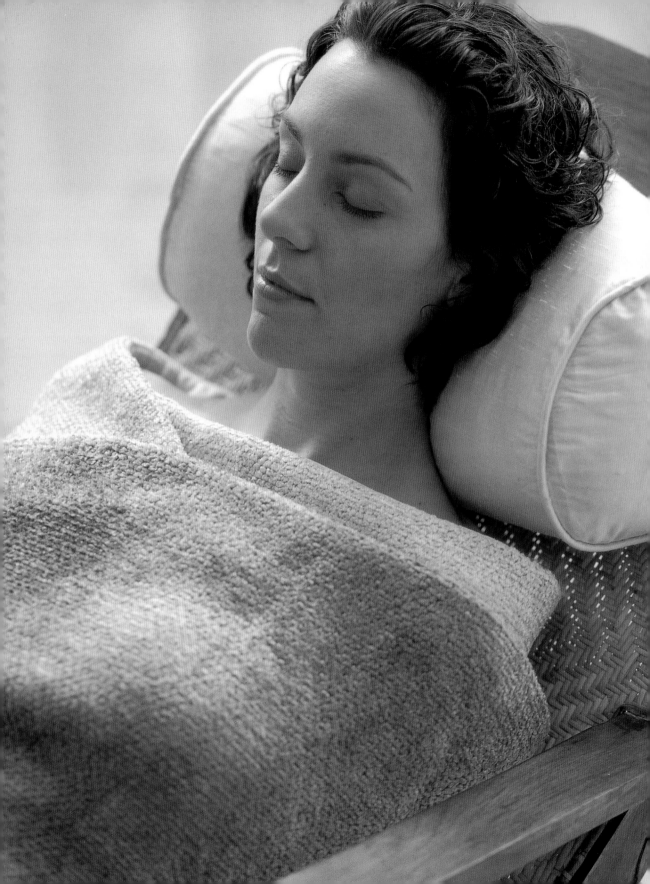

indulge

Part of being a grown-up is knowing what you enjoy—the food you like to savor, the company you prefer to keep, the activities you love to do. Sometimes, though, you might feel a little guilty about indulging in life's pleasures (we women tend to be programmed that way—after all, there's so much else to do!). But there's a time and a place for everything, and when it's your turn to revel in a little well-deserved pampering, we've got some ideas for you.

The activities you'll find in this chapter delight the senses—from making your bedroom smell delicious to exchanging massages with a loved one by a flickering fire. The skin-care and spa treatments go beyond simple maintenance; these are serious, thorough regimens that are well worth the time it takes to do them. You'll also find suggestions for revitalizing a tense, tired body, slowing down enough to reconnect with your surroundings, and surrendering to an adult version of time-out. Whatever activity you choose, remember this: An indulgence should please the senses, calm the mind, and lift the spirit. And, above all, it should make you happy.

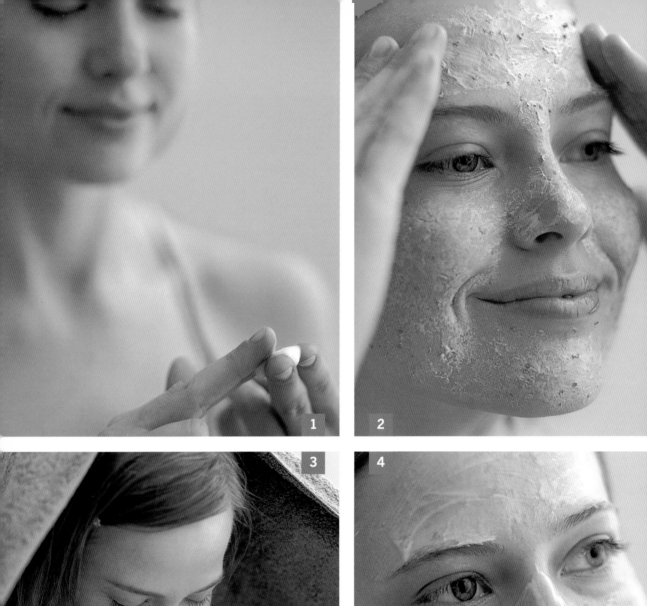

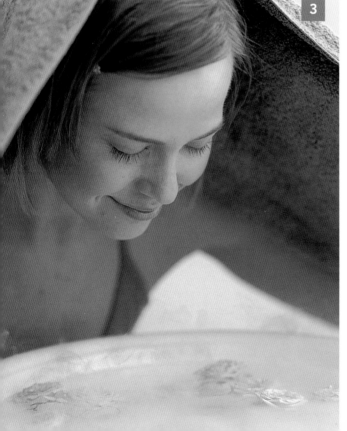

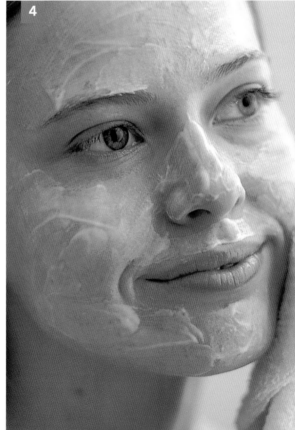

luxe facial

Good daily skin care is essential to maintaining its condition. Once a week or so, supplement your routine with a facial to enhance your healthy-looking glow.

1 As with any face-care regimen, begin by cleansing your face with a product appropriate for your skin type (see pages 54 and 56◄). Wet your face, and apply a thumbnail-size dollop of cleanser, using gentle, circular motions to massage it over your entire face and neck. Rinse with tepid water and pat your face and neck dry.

2 Next, exfoliate your skin to remove dead cells, impurities, and sebum (oil). Exfoliating speeds up cell renewal and allows a smooth, glowing new layer of skin to emerge. Again, it's important to use a gentle product formulated for your particular skin type. Lightly rub your fingers in circles over your face, taking care to avoid the eye area. Rinse thoroughly with tepid water and pat dry.

3 Fill a bowl with boiling water. Add a few drops of essential oil: If your skin is dry, a rose-and-frankincense blend is an excellent choice, while lavender works well for dry-to-normal skin, chamomile helps soothe sensitive skin, and lemon suits oily skin. Mix the oil and water well. Lean over the bowl, keeping your face ten to 12 inches away from the steaming water. Drape a bath towel over your head, creating a tent to trap the vapors. Steam your face for five to ten minutes.

4 While your skin is still damp from the steam, apply a facial mask formulated for your skin type and condition (for instance, a product that's highly moisturizing, purifying, or soothing). Spread a small amount over your face in a thin, even layer, and leave on for ten to 20 minutes. Remove the mask with a wet cloth and gently pat dry. Unless your skin is very oily, complete your luxurious facial by applying a moisturizing cream compatible with your skin type.

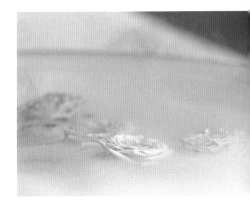

Rose to the Rescue
Cooling, relaxing, and toning (but very pricey in undiluted form), rose essential oil is celebrated for its rejuvenating effects, especially for dry or mature skin. It is used to soften wrinkles, moisturize, help reduce puffiness, and relieve clogged pores. In addition, its sweet floral aroma is quite soothing and helps promote restful sleep.

indulge

cat and cow

These satisfying yoga poses were inspired by the arc of a cat's back and a cow's swaybacked posture. Easy to do, they stretch your back and strengthen core muscles.

Give Yourself a Lift

Many people lift heavy objects incorrectly, which is one of the most common causes of back injury. When picking up a heavy object, be sure to squat down, tuck in your buttocks, and hold the object close to you. Keep your back straight, and rise using the muscles of your legs to power the lift—not your vulnerable back.

1 For the Cow pose, begin on all fours, with your palms positioned directly beneath your shoulders, your knees beneath your hips, and your elbows relaxed. (If you have weak or tender wrists, relieve the pressure on them by making fists, thumbs forward, with your hands on the floor.) Inhaling, press your belly down as your chest expands and gently lift your head and tailbone, lending a slight curve to your back, a bit reminiscent of a cow's swaybacked appearance.

2 For the Cat pose, exhale while contracting your diaphragm and abdomen, and lift your back as you lower your head and tailbone, like a cat engaged in a luxurious stretch.

Repeat the sequence for four to ten breaths. You might want to practice *mantra japa,* the repetition of a word or phrase. Done either silently or out loud and linked to coincide with the pace of your breathing, it can help you create a more meditative experience as you perform the poses. You may use any uplifting word or phrase. If none comes immediately to mind, try using the simple yet profound *shanti* (pronounced SHAHN-tee), which means "peace" in Sanskrit.

BABYING YOUR BACK

While back pain occurs all too easily among women, it's also easy to develop good habits that will help you ward it off. For instance, take frequent breaks to stretch when you work at a desk or computer. Here are some more do's and don'ts.

DO:	DON'T:
• Sleep on your side, with a pillow that supports your neck.	• Sleep on your stomach.
• Keep feet on the floor when sitting.	• Cross your legs when sitting.
• Use a chair with armrests.	• Carry a heavy purse, which causes your weight to shift to one side.
• Maintain good form when playing sports or doing housework.	• Wear high heels.
• Exercise your abs and back muscles.	• Slouch.
	• Lean into a mirror when grooming.

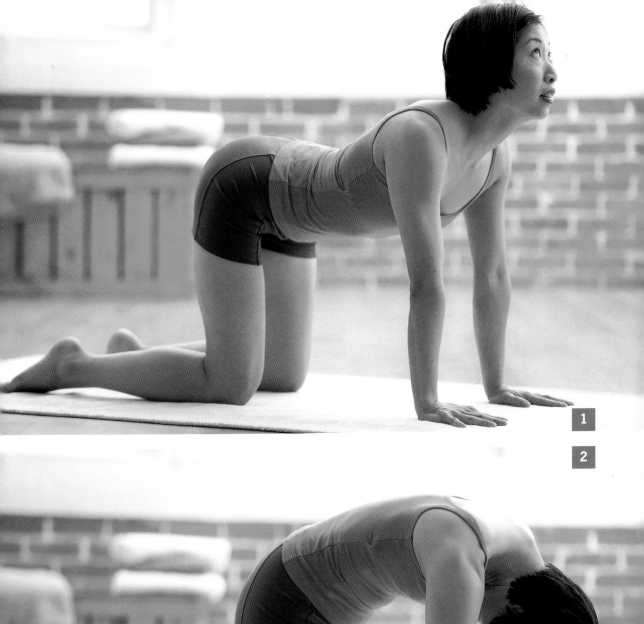

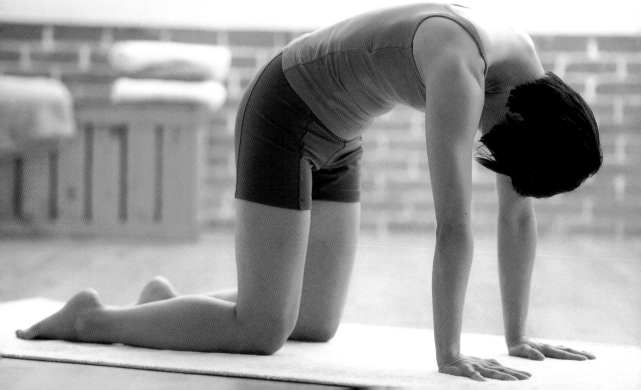

1

2

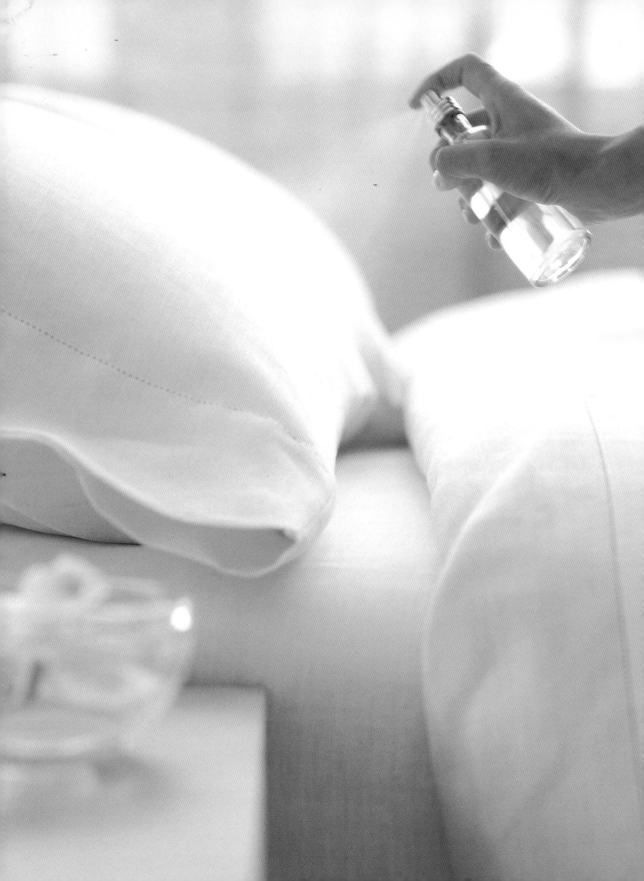

bedroom aromatherapy

Using essential oils in the bedroom can conjure up
associations of freshness, warmth, seduction, or peace—
whatever mood you'd like your special refuge to reflect.

As the room in which we sleep, dream, make love, and retreat, the
bedroom deserves extra attention and a dash of creativity. Decorating
it to your liking and keeping it clean and free of clutter is crucial to
making it feel like a place of refuge and indulgence. Helpful, too, is
infusing your bedroom with just the right aroma.

Misting essential oils throughout your bedroom is a delightful way
to create a mood. Just add a favorite essential oil or blend (see the
recipe at right) to a spray-mister filled with distilled water. Besides
spraying your mixture into the air, you can lightly spritz it on your
bed linens, drapes, and carpet. (Use light, clear oils to avoid stains,
and don't spray over wood furniture.) Choose a scent that suits your
needs: Bergamot or Roman chamomile may help reduce stress levels.
Lavender may help you relax. If romance is on your mind, ylang-
ylang's exotic floral fragrance is said to be an aphrodisiac, as are
patchouli and sandalwood. Use lemon or grapefruit oils to freshen
up the room; try eucalyptus to banish stale smells—and repel insects.

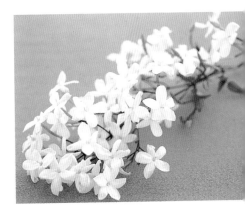

Indulgent Spray-Mister Blend

8 ounces distilled water

8 drops jasmine essential oil

7 drops lavender essential oil

7 drops sandalwood essential oil

3 drops vetiver essential oil

"NOT TONIGHT, JOSEPHINE"

No one really knows if Napoleon ever uttered these famous words
to his empress, but apparently Josephine had one boudoir habit
that greatly offended her husband. She reputedly was extremely
fond of musk and had her bedroom wallpaper impregnated with
its pungent, sensual scent. Alas, instead of stoking the fires of
desire in her husband, she succeeded only in giving him a throbbing
headache. In revenge, the emperor had her boudoir walls doused in
lime and showered Josephine with his own favorite perfume, made
from violets—flowers that he later had planted on her grave.

fireside massage

Exchanging massages by a warm, crackling fire can be a relaxing, romantic, and wonderfully nonverbal way to connect with your partner.

On a chilly evening, a blazing fireplace exerts a powerful primal attraction: The warmth is relaxing and comforting, the play of light and shadow is soothingly hypnotic, and the crackle and smoky smell awaken our senses. It is a perfect setting for practicing intimate touch. Snuggle up near the fireplace, and ask your partner to follow these instructions for a blissful massage. (If you're not too blissed out afterward, you might feel like reciprocating.)

1 Experiment with light, fast glides over the surface of the head, using gentle fingers to comb down through the hair. Begin the first strokes at the hairline on the forehead and sweep down to the ends. Then move back up to a different position at the hairline and repeat, until you've gently stroked the entire head.

2 Sometimes the perfect touch for relaxation is a light sweep across the skin. Using the flat of your palms and easy pressure, place your hands low on your partner's back and sweep up to the base of the neck. Then fan your hands out to the edge of the shoulders and sweep back down the sides, returning to the waist and lower back. Repeat this pattern, encouraging your partner to breathe deeply and let the cares of the world slip away with each stroke.

3 To help work out the tension that tends to accumulate between the shoulder blades, stabilize your partner with one hand on her shoulder. With your other hand, press and run your thumb into the muscles between the shoulder blades and spine. Follow the edge of each shoulder blade from top to bottom, gliding up and down. Start with gentle pressure and work more deeply as the muscles relax.

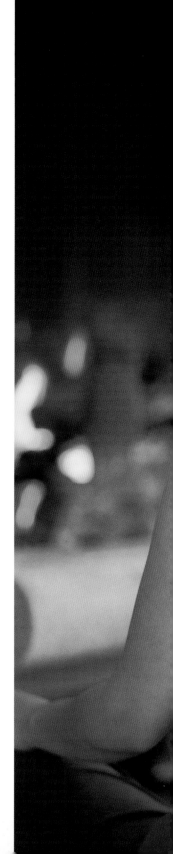

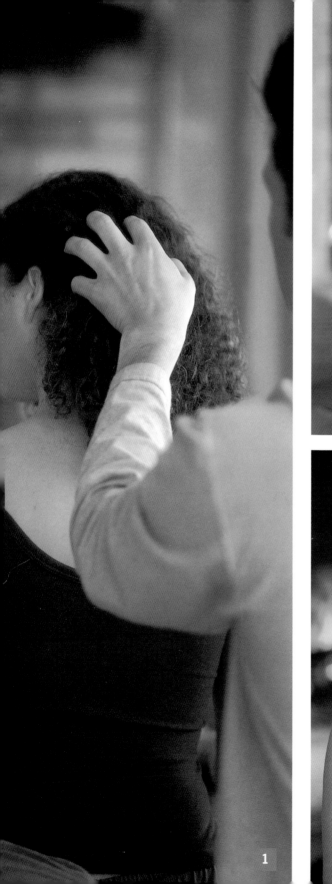
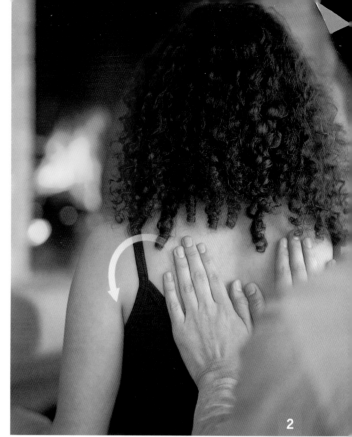
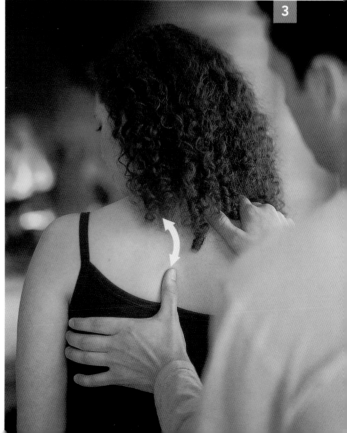

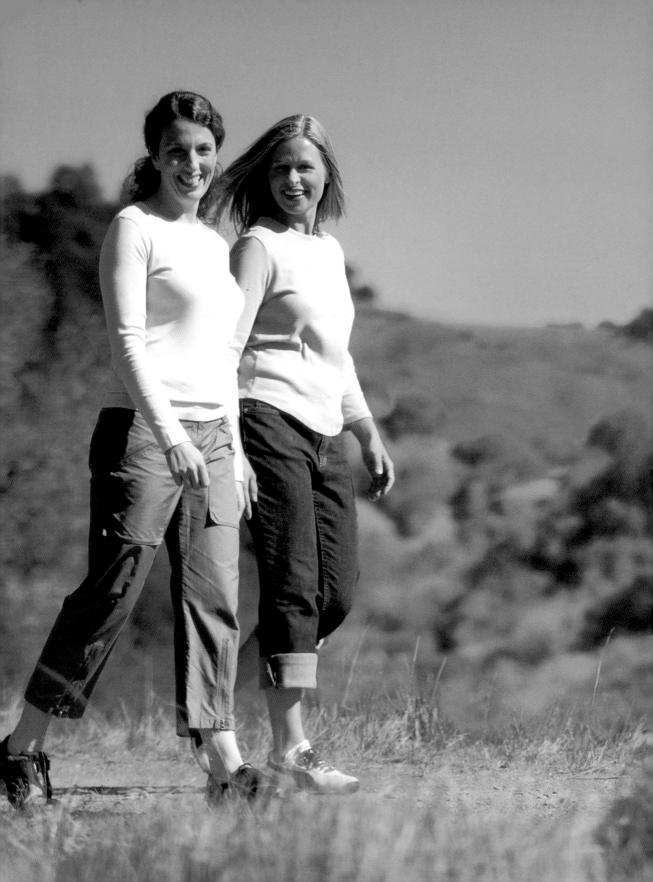

In many cultures, the act of walking has been reduced to a necessary evil, something we do when we can't find a convenient parking spot or have to trudge from the subway to the office. We don't have the time, we don't have the patience—heck, we often don't even have the right shoes. So it may seem strange to think of walking as an indulgence, but in today's rush-rush society, that's just what it can be. Not only is it an excellent and accessible form of exercise, it's a way to connect with your immediate environment, and it's a balm for the mind and soul.

the walking cure

Walking to work (or at least part of the way—get off the bus one stop earlier, for instance, or park a fair distance away) lets you collect your thoughts and rev up your body. And after a long day's toil, a walk provides a luxurious stretch for tight and restless limbs and helps work off tension and anxiety. Walking your children to school even one morning a week can be true quality time, an opportunity to talk, hold hands, and demonstrate how much you value their company. Going for a leisurely stroll lets you rediscover your own neighborhood—or discover a new one in an especially intimate, in-the-moment way. Invite along a friend and explore a nearby park or public garden; there's something about the slow pace, shared exercise, and being part of nature that fosters a sense of camaraderie and easy conversation. So go ahead—make time to walk, and stop and smell the roses. Maybe even literally.

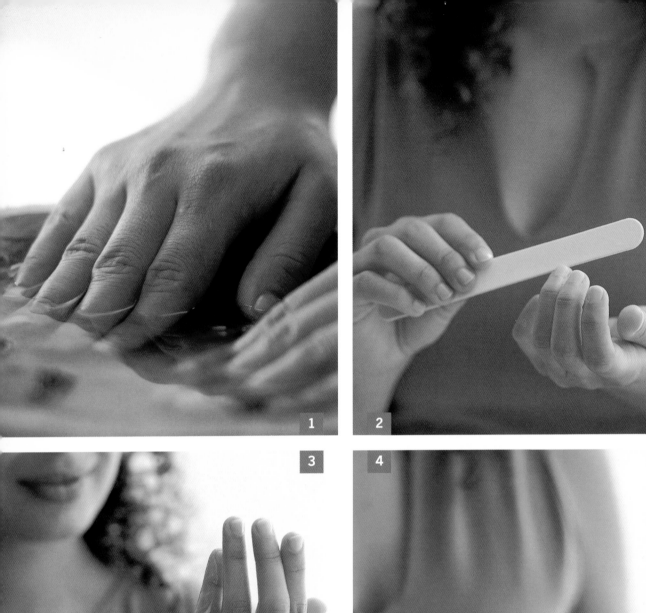

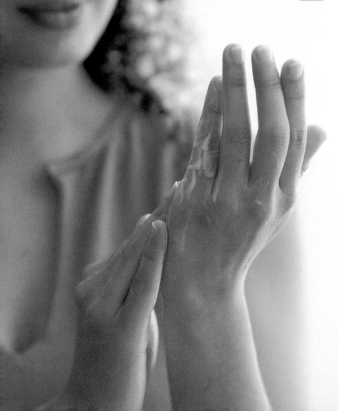

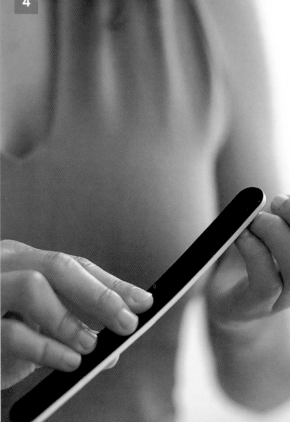

home manicure

Parched skin? Uneven or brittle nails? Unruly cuticles?
It's time to give your hardworking hands a little TLC with
a manicure designed to make them look and feel good.

1 Begin your manicure by filling a medium-size bowl with warm
water. Add two drops of lavender essential oil; the lavender acts as a
soothing, antibacterial agent, helping to clean and disinfect nail beds
(it smells wonderful, too). Immerse the tips of your fingers in the
water, ensuring that your nails and cuticles are completely covered.
Soak your fingers for at least five minutes to soften the cuticles and
prime your nails for the remaining steps.

2 Using an emery board, file each nail to form a pleasing shape and
eliminate any ragged edges. (Don't use a metal file; its harsh surface
can damage nails.) Start from one side and, in one smooth movement,
draw the file toward the center of the nail several times; then repeat
on the other side. Be careful not to saw back and forth—that causes
nails to splinter. After you've finished filing your nails, gently push
back the cuticles using an orange stick wrapped in a small piece of
cotton. (Although some professionals still do this, never cut your
cuticles, as cutting can increase the risk of an infection.) Following
the natural contours of your nails, try to expose as much of the nail
surface as possible to give each one a long, elegant silhouette.

3 Since your hands have fewer oil glands than the rest of your body,
they are prone to premature aging and feeling dry. Apply an intensive
restorative lotion, such as one containing vitamin E or hemp, to keep
them well hydrated. It's also important to use a daily sunscreen on
your hands to help keep wrinkles and age spots at bay.

4 Use a buffing file or block to give your nails a natural shine. Hold
the buffing tool between your thumb and fingers while you curl the
fingers of your other hand in toward your palm. Extend one finger at
a time, and apply the buffer in a back-and-forth motion across each
nail. Use quick, smooth strokes to give nails a healthy, polished look.

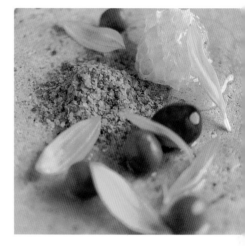

Intensive Care for Cuticles

If your cuticles are truly in sorry shape,
whip up an effective overnight treatment in
your kitchen. Just before bedtime, blend
one teaspoon of honey with one teaspoon
of sunflower, wheat germ, or olive oil in a
small bowl. Dip your fingers into the mix
and massage it into the beds of your nails
and cuticles. Cover your hands with cotton
gloves (or use a pair of soft cotton socks
as mittens) and leave on overnight.

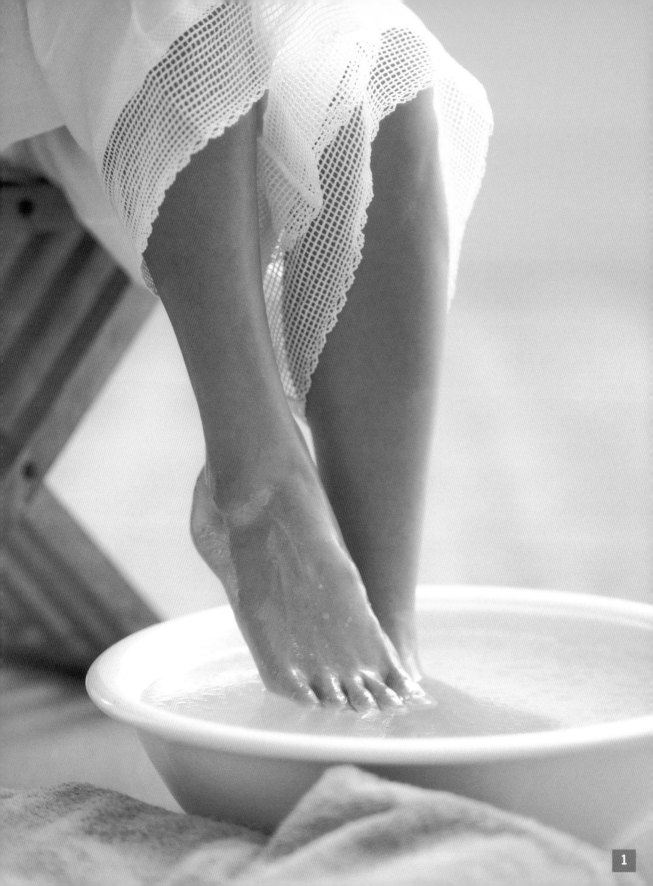

dry-feet hydration

A moisturizing soak, a little judicious heel-filing, and
an overnight hydrating treatment can work wonders
on your feet if they tend to be dry or rough.

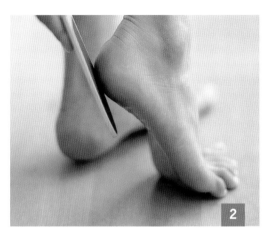

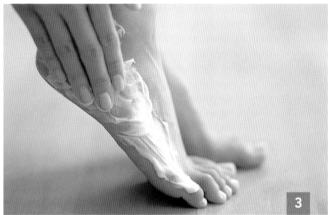

1 Fill a bowl large enough to immerse your feet completely with
warm water, then add five drops of neroli essential oil and three
tablespoons of olive oil and mix well. Neroli's floral fragrance is
relaxing and uplifting; olive oil is known for its softening, emollient
properties. Soak your feet for 15 minutes, then rest them on a towel.

2 While your feet are still damp, using a firm back-and-forth motion
with a foot file, remove the dead skin that tends to accumulate on
the heels, balls of the feet, and bottoms of big toes. Check every few
strokes to feel your skin; when it no longer feels rough in a certain
area, move on to the next problem spot. (And, of course, stop at any
sign of pain.) If your feet are severely dry and cracked, it might take
several treatments to smooth them, so don't expect instant miracles.

3 Hydrate your newly exposed fresh skin. For dramatic results, slather
your feet with a shea-butter balm or other intensive moisturizer such
as hemp oil, then slip on a pair of deep-moisturizing foot booties (or
cotton socks) and leave them on overnight.

The Skinny on Shoes
Many women have a love affair with
shoes, but these delightful and
necessary accessories are to blame
for many foot problems. Pointed
toes, high heels, a lack of proper
padding, and poor fit contribute to
everything from bunions to corns,
calluses to acute pain (and not just
in our feet—backs suffer, too, when
we prance about in high heels).

deep conditioning

Treating hair with a warm oil base containing essential oils promotes shine and strength, helping combat the effects of blow-drying, sunlight, and chemical processes.

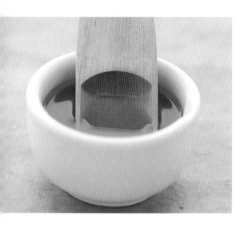

Deep-Conditioning Hair Treatment

1 teaspoon Brazil nut oil

1 teaspoon olive oil

1 teaspoon sesame oil

½ teaspoon honey

2 drops geranium essential oil

2 drops lavender essential oil

1 Mix the ingredients in the recipe at left in a small bowl or plastic bottle. Warm the oil mixture by setting the container in a large bowl or pan of hot water for a few minutes. (Heated oils can penetrate your hair better than unheated ones, making them more effective.)

2 After wetting your hair, rub the oil on your fingers and work it through your hair, starting at the top and moving down to the ends.

3 Soak a towel in warm water and wring it out. (Or put a damp towel in your dryer for a few minutes to warm it.) Wrap the towel around your hair. Leave it on for five to 15 minutes. (One of the advantages of a longer conditioning treatment is that it gives you time to take a relaxing bath, meditate, sit outdoors, or read a book.) Then wash your hair with your regular shampoo.

4 Comb your hair with a broad-toothed comb (brushes can break wet hair strands). Indulge in this treatment every few weeks—more often if your hair is very dry or damaged, less often if it's oily or fine.

A HAIR-RAISING STORY

Like nails, feathers, and even the baleen of whales, hair is a form of protein known as keratin. Human hair is strong—as strong as an iron wire, by some accounts—but it can be damaged by chemical treatments, blow drying, sunlight, chlorine, and rough handling. Badly damaged hair might never recover—you'll have to wait for the old hair to fall out of its follicle and be replaced by new hair—but conditioning can help the *appearance* of your hair. That's because damaged hair tends to have ruffled scales, and conditioners smooth those scales down, thus creating a smooth, shiny look.

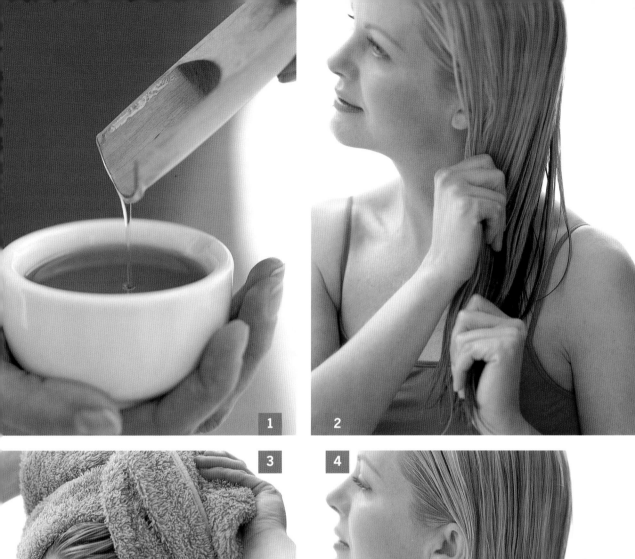
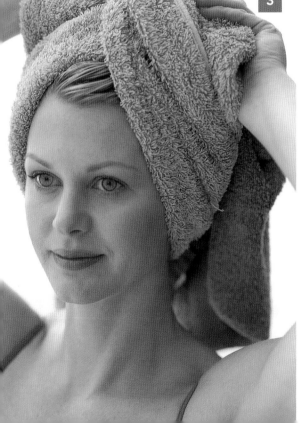
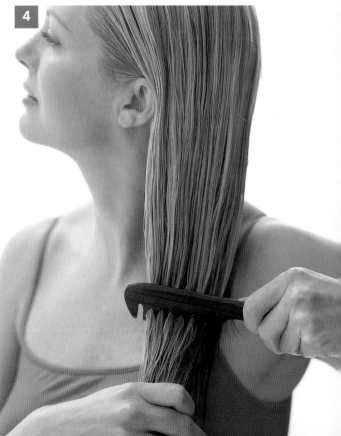

restful wrap

After a bath or simply when you're in need of some serious downtime, resting in a nest of soft, warm blankets can make you feel pampered and restored.

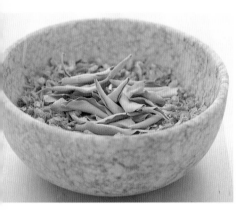

Restful Wrap Spray-Mister Blend

1 cup distilled water

2 drops jasmine essential oil

1 drop clary sage essential oil

Surrendering to Serenity

According to aromatherapists, clary sage (the dried leaves pictured above) can be a potent antidote to depression and anxiety, and is something of an aphrodisiac. Jasmine (the dried flowers above) also has long been thought to relieve anxiety, stress, and depression, as well as bolster the libido.

Topping off an at-home bath ritual (see page 205 ◄) with a period of rest under warm blankets is often considered the most important step of all. (Bath or no bath, a restful wrap isn't a bad escape any time you need a little quiet cocooning time.) During this rest period, your parasympathetic nervous system works its restorative magic, helping to slow down your heart rate, regulate the digestion of food, and otherwise help your body run more smoothly and efficiently.

To prepare for your restful wrap, spread two or three heavy blankets on your bed; use a soft blanket on top, as it will be the layer in contact with your body. Place one or two pillows on the bed, so you can rest your head at a comfortable height and angle. Remove all your clothing and lie on the blankets, wrapping them snugly around your body. Rest with your eyes closed for 20 to 30 minutes. Use the time to meditate, remember the positive events of the day, fantasize about your next vacation—anything but worry.

For an indulgent variation on the above, use a spray-mister to scent the blankets used in your wrap with your favorite essential oils (see our suggestion for a restful blend at left). If you prefer, you could just spray a bath towel with the essential-oil blend and place that on top of the blankets instead (it's easier to wash the scent out of a towel than a pile of blankets). In cool weather, you also can heat up your wrap by spraying a little water on your bath towel or the top blanket and tumbling it in the dryer for about ten minutes right before you place it on the bed. To make the soothing heat last even longer, place a hot-water bottle or heating pad in the wrap.

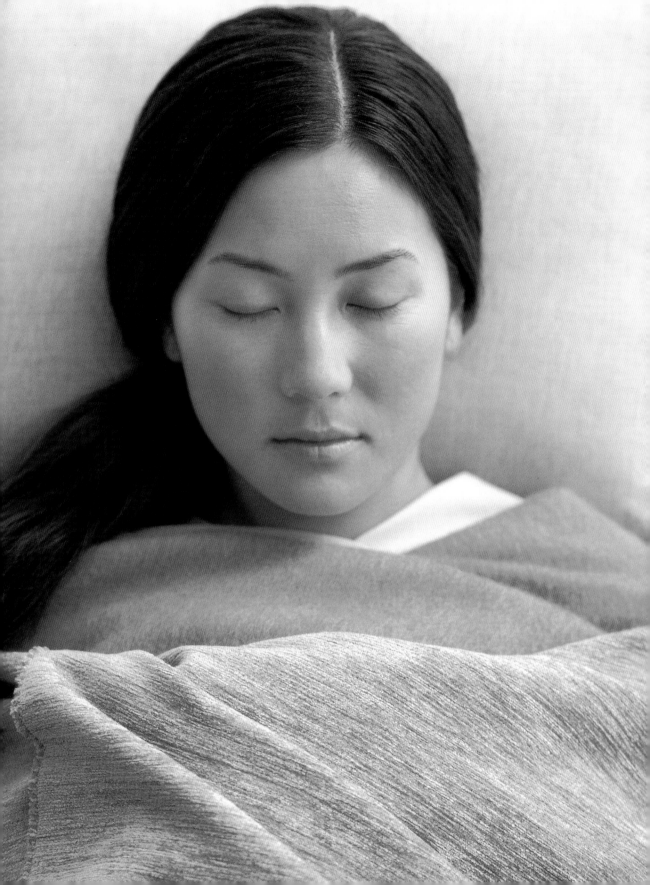

chilled rhubarb soup

Ideally made with the lovely red stalks of fresh rhubarb, this light and refreshing dessert tastes decadently rich but is surprisingly low in fat and calories.

Ingredients

2 cups fresh rhubarb, cut into ½-inch slices (or 10 ounces frozen rhubarb)

1 cup thinly sliced strawberries, plus a few reserved for garnish

1½ cups water

½ cup orange juice

⅓ cup sugar

2 teaspoons finely grated orange zest

2 tablespoons Triple Sec liqueur

Crème fraîche or vanilla yogurt (optional)

- Serves: 4
- Prep time: 10 minutes
- Cook time: 10 minutes, plus 2 hours chilling time

Chilled dessert soups lend a touch of sweetness and sophistication to a summer night's supper. This rhubarb soup can be made the day ahead and stored in the refrigerator until it's time for dessert. Show off its lovely rosy color by serving the soup in small glass bowls. A few sliced strawberries make an attractive garnish, and, if you like, you can top it all off with a dollop of crème fraîche or yogurt.

1 In a medium saucepan, combine the rhubarb and strawberries with the water, orange juice, and sugar. Bring to a boil, lower heat, and simmer for ten to 12 minutes, stirring occasionally, until the rhubarb and strawberries are very soft.

2 Remove the pan from the heat; add the orange zest and Triple Sec liqueur. Using a wire whisk, stir the rhubarb mixture to break up the coarse pieces of rhubarb and strawberries.

3 Pour into a bowl, cover, and refrigerate for at least two hours before serving. Top servings with crème fraîche or yogurt, if desired.

Nutritional Information Per Serving

Here's one rich-tasting dessert that is free of both fat and cholesterol.

Calories	120
Kilojoules	502
Protein	1 g
Carbohydrates	28 g
Total Fat	0.5 g
Saturated Fat	0 g
Cholesterol	0 mg
Sodium	5 mg
Dietary Fiber	1 g

HEART-HEALTHY RHUBARB

Both slightly sweet and slightly sour, rhubarb is a lovely, complex ingredient for pies, jams, sauces, and other culinary creations. This red-stalked vegetable is also good for your heart. One Canadian study found that when men with very high levels of cholesterol ate powdered dietary fiber from rhubarb, their LDL (or bad) cholesterol levels dropped between 9 and 20 percent. Another health benefit: Rhubarb has a fair amount of potassium and vitamin C. (However, its leaves and roots are toxic, so be sure to eat only the stalks.)

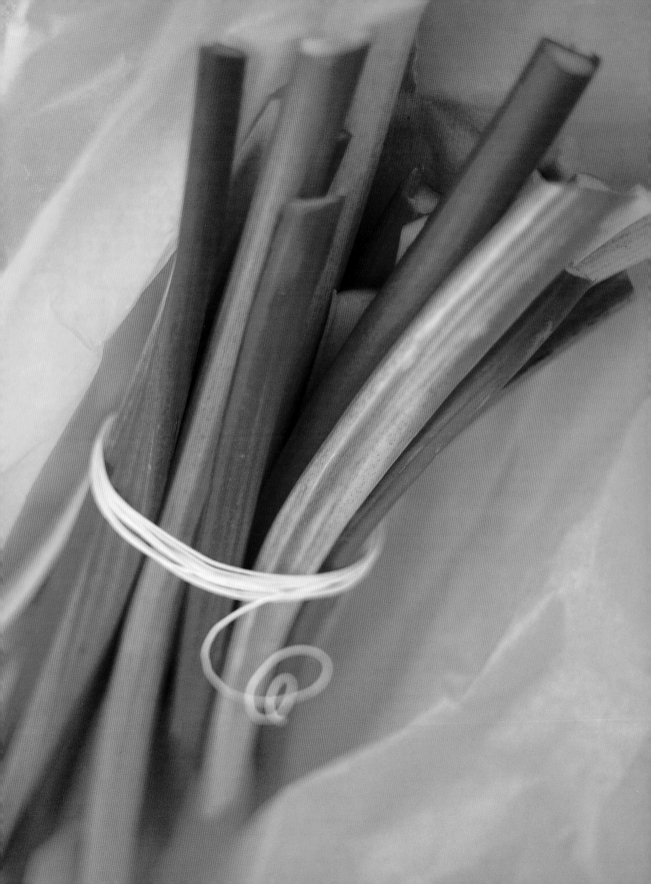

explore

Routines are comfortable. Routines streamline our days. Routines steer us to the tried and true. And routines can be boring. Time to see what else might be waiting for us out there…

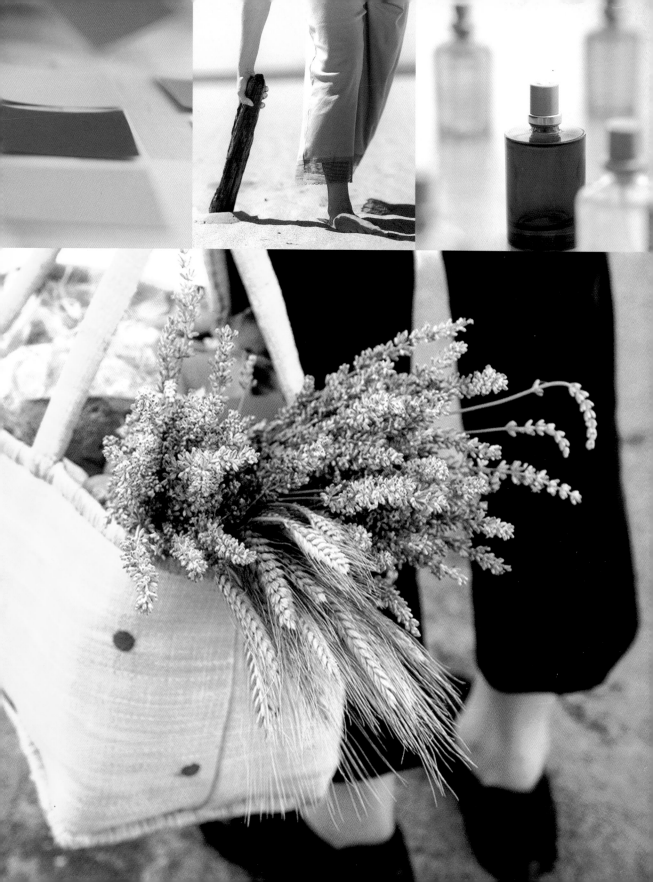

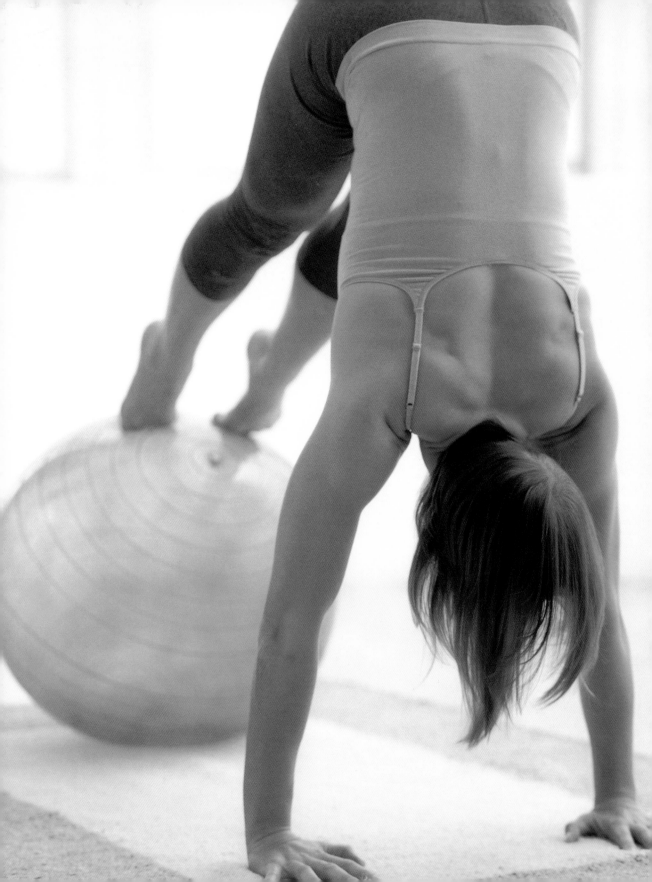

explore

To one degree or another, we are all creatures of habit, which is not necessarily a bad thing. Routines are the fruit of our past experiences, and they are important. They bring order to chaos, make us more efficient, and create a sense of consistency in what can be an alarmingly unpredictable world. But sometimes what seems like a cozy routine is actually a rut—a set of habits so deeply ingrained you'd need a team of plow horses to pull you out.

Well, we can't harness those horses, but we can toss you a few lifelines in the form of fresh ideas. You don't need to do anything really drastic; basically, it's just a matter of putting a new twist on a familiar favorite. Love to cook but find yourself sticking to the same tired repertoire of recipes? Try exploring farmers' markets, natural food stores, or ethnic groceries for some culinary inspiration. Exercise routine getting a little stale? The answer just may be a gym class away. Feeling restless during your meditation sessions? You might experiment with the ways color can affect your perceptions of the world or try to unlock a labyrinth's twisting mysteries. Whatever your quest, and whatever path you take to get there, exploring is sure to enrich your body and soul—and keep life interesting.

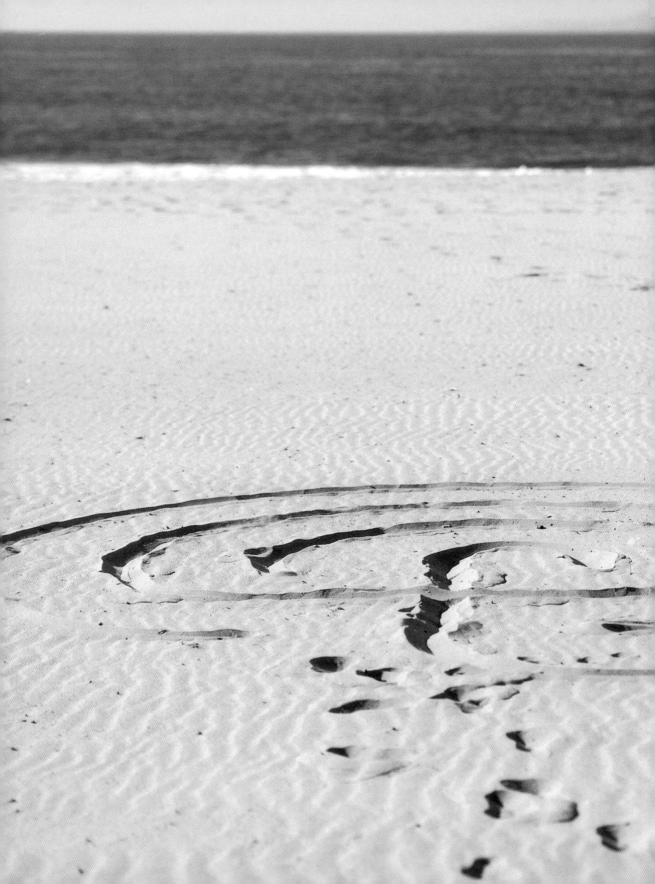

learning from labyrinths

Create your own labyrinth by drawing a classical figure in the sand and following its twists and curves to a calmer and more contemplative state of mind.

Humans have been creating labyrinths—walking paths that spiral back on themselves—for thousands of years. The ancient Greeks, Native Americans, and Mayans all used labyrinths in sacred rituals. Medieval Europeans created elaborate labyrinths for many of their churches; the French installed one of the most famous ones, fashioned of inlaid marble, at Chartres Cathedral in the 13th century. The designs and materials used may have varied greatly, but they all served as profound symbols of life, death, and mystery, a way to journey to one's own center and then out into the world again.

Today, churches, parks, medical centers, spas, and schools—even a few jails—offer labyrinths for the public to wander. Whether you see them as symbolic of life's journey, paths to salvation, metaphors for finding your own spiritual track, or intriguing vehicles for meditation, labyrinths can help you quiet your mind and find solace. If one isn't available in your area (or you're just the do-it-yourself type), you can make your own simple labyrinth in the sand or dirt; the fact that it's a small labyrinth doesn't make it any less spiritual.

DON'T CALL IT A MAZE

Labyrinth aficionados bristle when one of their beloved paths is called a maze. Mazes, they point out, can have several entrances and paths, often don't lead to a center, and contain dead ends. Labyrinths have only one path; while it might twist and turn, it's simple to follow and a sojourner won't ever get lost. There are no dead ends or wrong turns. As Lauren Artress, creator of The Worldwide Labyrinth Project, explains: "A labyrinth is designed for you to find your way. A maze is designed for you to lose your way."

step-by-step sequence ▶

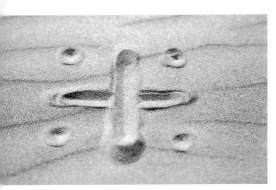

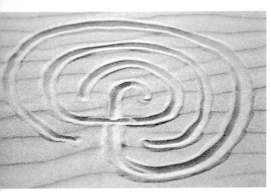

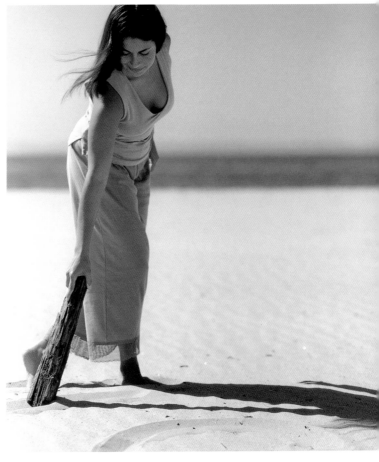

1 To create a classical labyrinth, draw a cross about six feet wide and place a dot in each quadrant. Next, draw four curving, clockwise lines in the following order: join the top of the cross to the top right dot; next, connect the top left dot to the right arm of the cross; then join the left arm of the cross to the bottom right dot; finally, circle from the bottom left dot all the way around to the bottom arm of the cross.

2 As you draw, try to have a calm, reflective spirit. Listen to the swish of the stick as it moves through the soft sand. Feel the warm touch of the sun on your skin. Try to move and breathe with focus and deliberation. Remember that the very act of making the labyrinth can be a type of moving meditation.

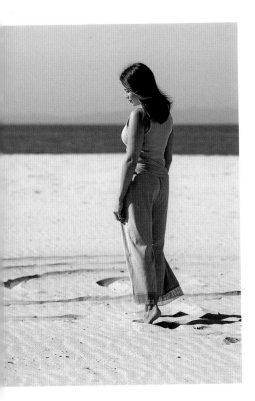

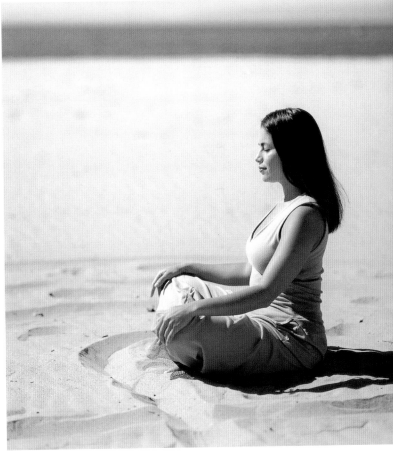

3 When you've finished, take a deep breath at the entrance of the labyrinth and clear your mind. Acknowledge the journey you are about to begin; you may even want to formalize this by bowing, saying a little prayer, or simply closing your eyes for a moment. Choose an intention for your walk, whether it's spiritual, reflective, or playful.

4 Follow the path toward the center of the labyrinth. Keep your mind quiet; let go of random thoughts and worries as they arise. Concentrate on putting one foot in front of the other and breathing regularly. When you reach the center, sit and spend some time meditating. (You may ponder a certain question or just want to sit quietly.) When you are ready to leave, follow your path out of the labyrinth, taking your insights with you.

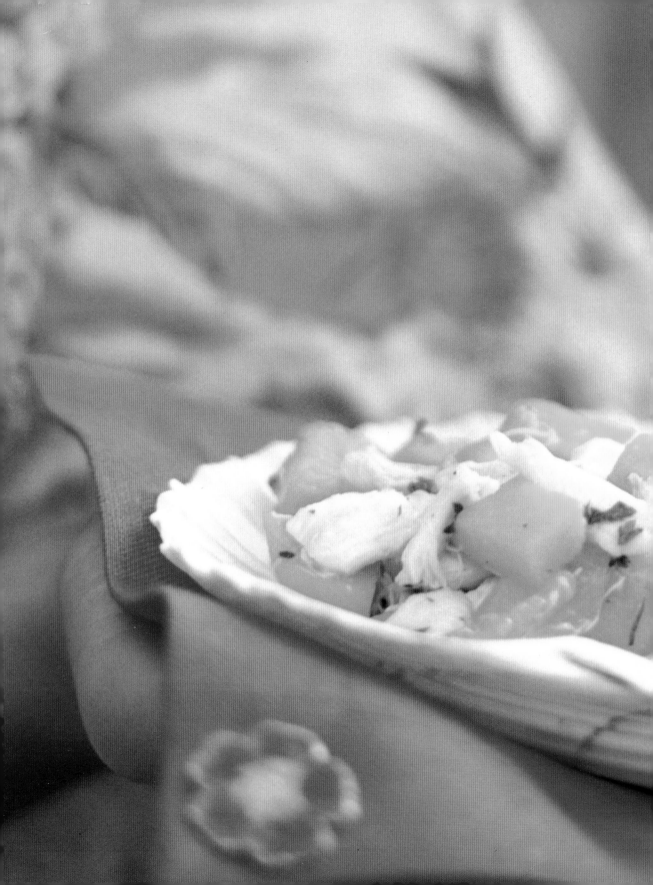

One enjoyable way to seek fresh culinary inspiration is by visiting farmers' markets, ethnic food stores, or purveyors of natural foods. You'll be exposed to a bounty of gorgeous fruits and vegetables; new and interesting types of meats, poultry, and fish; and freshly made cheeses and just-baked breads. Specialty stores such as butchers, fishmongers, and cheese shops often offer selections you can't find at a typical supermarket. As you stroll among the stalls or aisles, be sure to take some time to talk to the growers and proprietors; they're usually proud of their wares and happy to offer advice on selection and food preparation.

new food horizons

Cooking classes also can inspire you to explore a new ethnic cuisine or way of cooking. Besides formal cooking schools, establishments such as colleges, local recreation departments, cookware stores, supermarkets, restaurants, and wineries may hold classes in your area. Some offer cooking demonstrations, others specialize in hands-on classes, so you can choose the level of involvement you want. Of course, these days the Internet also makes it easy to find recipes and nutritional information for everything from anchovies to zucchini. Finally, don't forget the simplest standby: cooking magazines and cookbooks. Classic or new, general or specialized, these sources offer a wealth of new ideas for recipes, menus, entertaining, and food preparation.

color therapy

When you're feeling out of sorts, depressed, listless, or angry, color can brighten your mood. Color therapists even say that it can heal you when you're sick.

A Vision in Violet
A firm believer in the potency of color, Leonardo da Vinci reputedly basked in the glow of a violet stained-glass window to increase his creative powers. Try to achieve a similar effect by saturating your environment—from the clothing you wear to the color of your walls, for instance—with violet.

Color therapy, or chromotherapy, is a way of using color to treat or prevent mental and physical illnesses. Proponents of this theory reason that colors, which are a form of electromagnetic radiation, can affect the energy emitted by the various organs of the body, and have profound psychological effects as well. Chromotherapists might prescribe green for ulcers or yellow for depression, for example. You take your chromatic medicine in a variety of ways, ranging from installing a colored light bulb to eating foods of a particular hue.

Even scientists who scoff at chromotherapy recognize that color has a significant impact on the human psyche and can cause certain physiological reactions. People in a room painted in a cool color, such as a grayish blue, will crank up the thermostat higher than those in a yellow- or orange-colored room to feel warm. Altering the natural color of a food can make tasters turn against a dish they normally like—or even make them feel ill. And researchers have confirmed that colors influence people's moods: Some hues generally have a calming effect, while others prove cheerful or stimulating.

DO YOU CRAVE A COLOR?

When we're drawn to certain colors at a particular time, color therapists assert that we're lacking in the energy produced by that color. To see what hue your mind and body might be craving, scan the color bar at right. After a few moments, you're likely to gravitate to one color over the others.

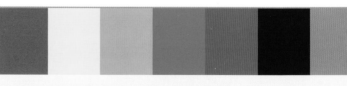

If you chose red, you're in need of energy or confidence. Yellow means you'd like to lighten a despondent mood. If you were drawn to orange, you crave mental energy and a sense of cheerfulness. Green means your nerves are frazzled and you feel off-balance emotionally. Blue helps you feel more serene and reflective. Indigo taps into your powers of intuition and alleviates frustration and fear. Violet makes you feel more creative and spiritual.

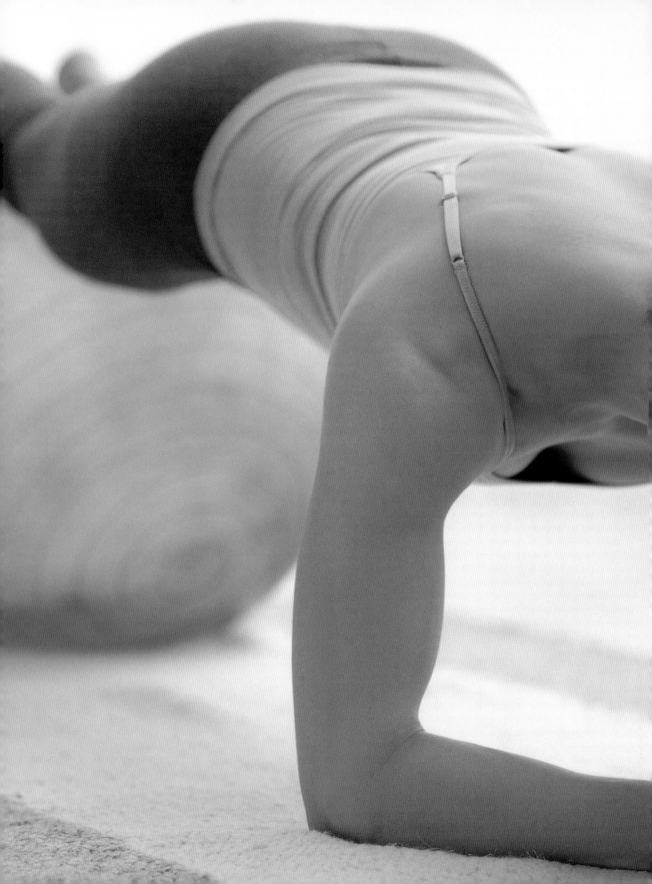

fitness ball

A staple in Pilates exercises, the use of a large, inflatable ball can help develop muscles that don't normally get challenged even in the most rigorous sports or classes.

Rolling around on a large ball may seem like child's play. But done correctly, ball work can be incredibly challenging as it helps you develop core muscles (see page 93 ◄) and a moment-to-moment balance that most floor exercises don't require. Using a ball also lets you do Pilates strengthening and stretching exercises that would otherwise require expensive equipment. Together, the ball and the Pilates tradition can help you align your body and strengthen your torso, both of which contribute to the long, lean physique that's characteristic of those who regularly practice Pilates.

You can buy a 55- to 65-centimeter fitness ball at almost any store that sells exercise equipment. (Generally people under five-foot-eight will be most comfortable with a 55-centimeter ball.) It helps to use the ball on a carpet—or, even better, a sticky yoga mat—so the ball doesn't slip around too much. Be sure to choose a real fitness ball as opposed to, say, a child's inflatable ball. Fitness balls are made to withstand more pressure and movement.

HAVING A BALL EXERCISING

Researchers from the University of Waterloo in Ontario, Canada, compared the rate of muscle activity doing curl-ups on the floor, a wobble board (a type of balance board), and a fitness ball. They found that the fitness ball afforded a much better workout than the flat surfaces; the fitness ball worked the upper abdominal muscles 25 percent harder, the lower abs 34 percent harder, and the external obliques (the group of muscles on the sides of the torso) 16 percent harder. Clearly, the muscles had to work harder to maintain balance on the unstable surface of the ball than on the flat surfaces.

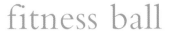

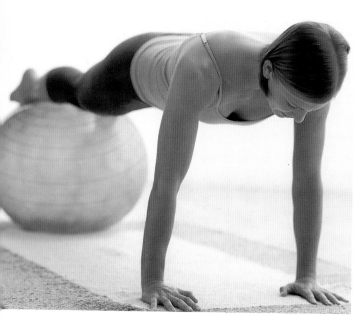

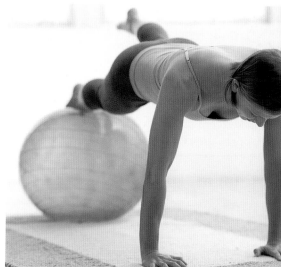

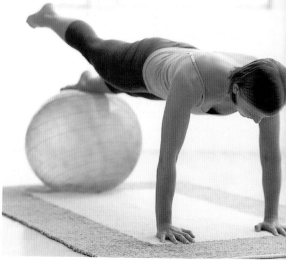

1 Start by balancing in a push-up position with your arms on the floor, fingers pointing forward, and the tops of your feet on the ball. Push your shoulder blades away from your spine and pull your ribs up, drawing in your abdominal muscles and tightening your buttocks. Avoid arching your back or letting your waist sag. Keep your neck straight and your eyes focused on the floor.

2 Lift one leg up, elongating your leg as much as possible and pointing your toes. Again, avoid arching your back or pushing your bottom up into the air. Maintain a level pelvis and draw your abs in.

3 Now work your other leg. Continue to alternate exercising your legs, lifting each one five to ten times. When you have finished, dismount carefully from the ball by bending your knees and bringing one leg down to the floor at a time.

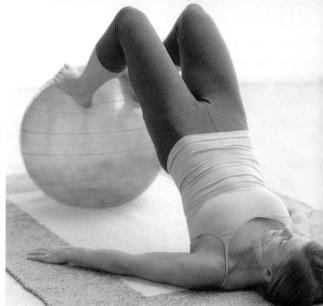

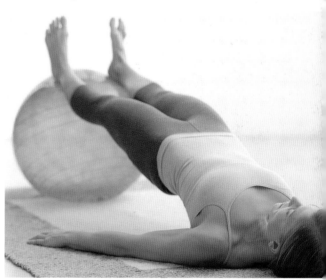

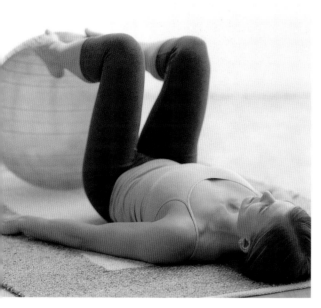

4 To start the next exercise, lie on your back and put your feet on the ball so that your knees are at a 90-degree angle and your hands are out to the side, palms down. Keep your abs pulled in, so your rib cage is pressed downward, toward the floor.

5 Push up on the ball with the bottoms of your feet, bend your knees, and rest on your shoulder blades. Avoid rolling back onto your neck.

6 Pushing the ball away from you, extend your knees so that your body forms a straight line. Rest your heels on the ball, and try to keep your hips up. Draw the ball toward you. Pressing down with the soles of your feet, lower your pelvis to the floor. Repeat Steps 4 through 6 eight times.

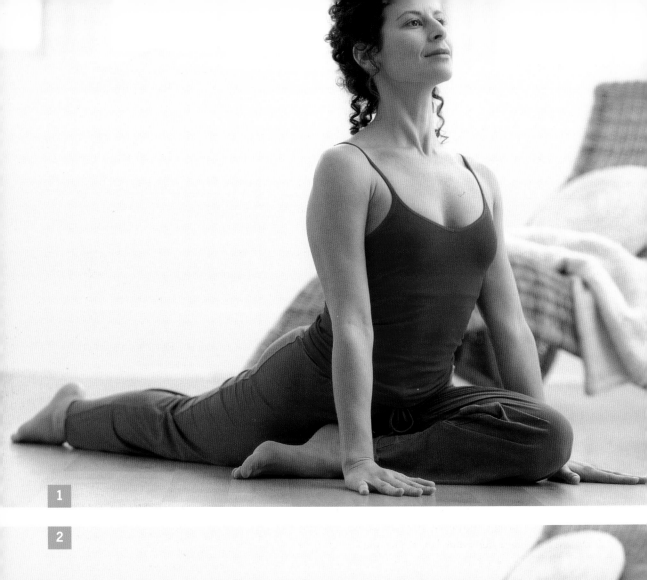

1

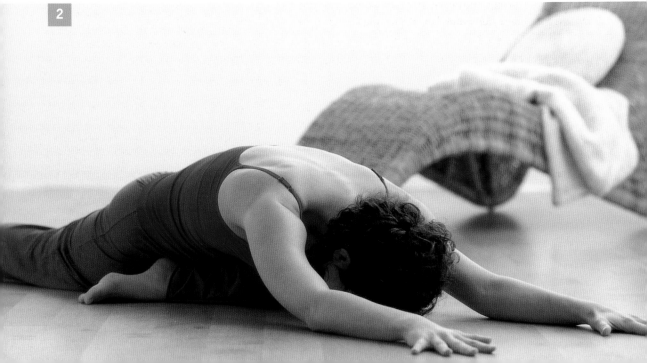

2

pigeon variations

Keep your yoga routine fresh and your body and mind stimulated by expanding your repertoire. Pigeon poses let you work with challenging but gratifying hip releases.

1 To perform the Pigeon pose, get on all fours. Bring your left knee forward between your hands, with your foot positioned to the right so your leg forms an inverted V shape. Extend your right leg back and allow your hips to sink, keeping them level to the floor. Be careful not to roll onto your left thigh or strain your knees. Elongate your spine, lift your chest, and keep your palms on the floor and your shoulders loose and low. Hold for four to six breaths (but release at the first sign of any strain). To release, push down with your palms, lift your hips, and slide your left leg back. Repeat on the other side.

2 In the Low Pigeon pose, your weight falls more on your arms and a bit less on your hips. From the Pigeon pose, relax over your bent leg. Lower your weight onto your forearms, placing them on the floor shoulder-width apart. If this is comfortable, release more weight onto your bent leg by extending your arms completely and letting your head rest on (or hang toward) the floor. Note any resistance in your body, and encourage these muscles to surrender to the pose. Hold for four to six breaths. Release and repeat on the other side. (For another hip-releasing pose, try Rock the Baby; see page 202 ◄.)

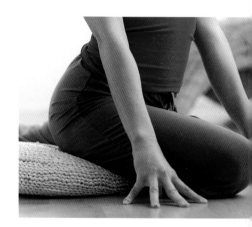

Get a Boost

If you find it difficult to keep your hips level in either Pigeon pose, try placing a firm pillow or a folded blanket under the hip of your bent-leg side. The farther your hips are from the floor, of course, the thicker the pillow or blanket needs to be. With regular practice, you gradually will need less support.

DIFFERENT TYPES OF HATHA YOGA

The poses and breathing exercises described in this book are in the tradition of Hatha yoga and are appropriate for beginners. But there are many varieties of Hatha yoga— some more challenging than others.

TYPE OF YOGA	PRIMARY CHARACTERISTICS
Ashtanga	A fast-paced sequence of poses requiring strict breath control
Bikram	A prescribed series of poses done in a room heated to about 105 degrees Fahrenheit with about 60 percent humidity
Jivamukti	Physically challenging yoga poses combined with a strong spiritual component
Sivananda	Practice of poses and breathing exercises, along with a vegetarian diet, meditation, positive thinking, and relaxation

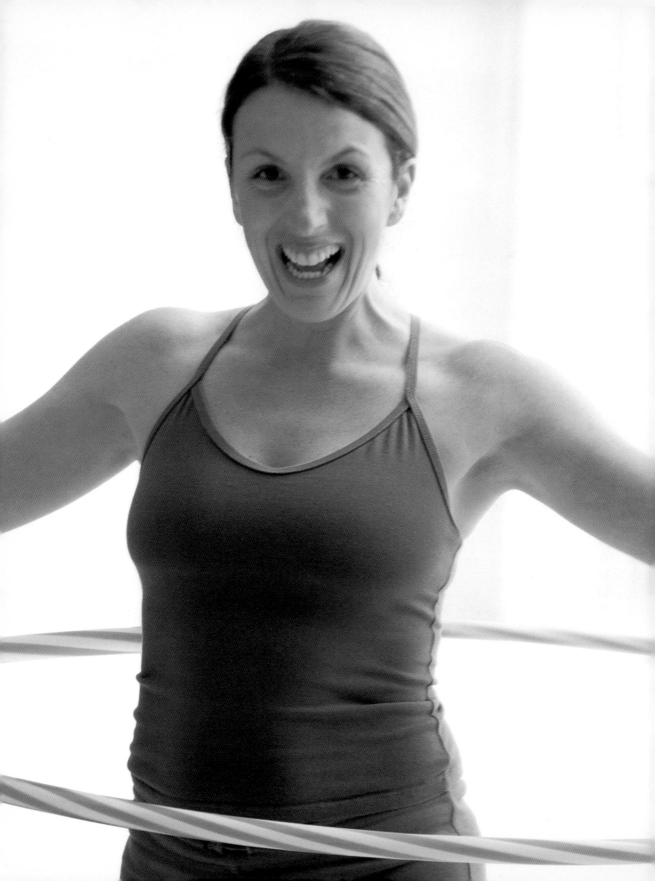

We run, we bike, we step, we hike—at some point, we find exercise routines that seem to work for our bodies, schedules, and skill sets. Unfortunately, many of us stay with these same old routines even when our minds and bodies might be craving something new.

shake up your routine

Exploring different athletic activities can alleviate the boredom that can sabotage even a committed exerciser, as well as help you strengthen other muscles, develop new kinds of coordination, and enhance your flexibility. Books and videos offer starting points, but classes will give you the benefit of an experienced instructor, who will coach you on proper form (which is critical to maximizing benefits as well as avoiding injuries), urge you on when you feel uninspired, and provide guidance if you encounter any difficulties. Look for someone who is knowledgeable and enthusiastic and who makes the class fun as well as challenging.

There are plenty of classes—with plenty of health benefits—from which to choose. A salsa class might help you get some rhythm. A step class can kick your cardiovascular system into action. A yoga class will help your balance, posture, and concentration. You might be surprised at the number of offerings—everything from hula-hooping to belly-dancing, jumping rope to aquatic tai chi.

Where to find new active things to do? In addition to health clubs and city recreational departments, check out local colleges, bulletin boards at sporting goods stores, and dance and yoga studios. If you're feeling shy or nervous, ask a friend to join you—your exercise time will become valuable friendship time, as well.

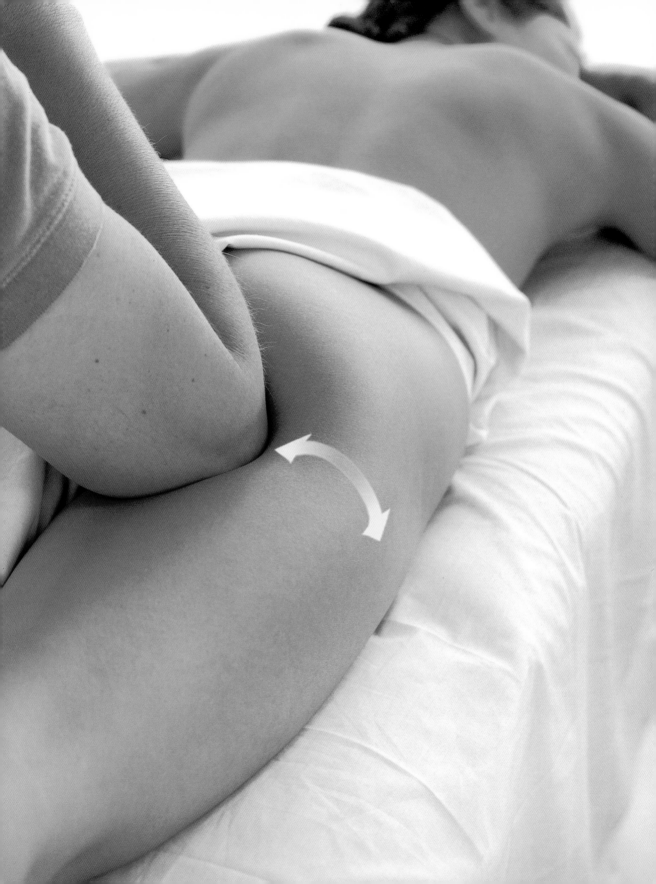

glute massage

Even women who routinely get massages might consider certain body parts off-limits. But sometimes pushing your comfort zone can yield unexpected pleasures.

Often, even professional full-body massages fail to include massaging the buttocks. Which is a shame, since we tend to carry a lot of tension in these muscles (the *glutei maximi*), the thickest in our bodies. So break out of the massage rut and trade glute massages with a friend or your partner. It will release pent-up tension, help tone the buttocks, and might even help break up cellulite by improving circulation and flushing out toxins. Besides, a glute massage just feels really, really good. Here are the steps for your massage partner to follow:

To begin, position one of your elbows at the bottom of one of the gluteal muscles. Using firm pressure, glide up alongside the tailbone to the thick muscles of the glutes. Then zigzag slowly back and forth across the muscles, working from the edge of the tailbone out to the wide part of the outer thigh and back in again. You'll know you're doing your job when you feel the fibers starting to separate. (See "When Good Fibers Go Bad" on page 126 ◄ for more information about the benefits of cross-fiber massage.)

Giving a cross-fiber massage can feel as if you are popping across taut ropes, but don't worry—this will help relax and soften the fibers. Soreness is common during and after cross-fiber work, but be careful not to overdo it. Excessive friction can injure the tissue. The rule of thumb: The deeper you go, the slower you go. Massage the muscles this way for about two to three minutes.

Now position yourself to one side of your friend and press your fingertips into the far side of the opposite gluteal muscle. Leaning back, pull toward the tailbone with alternating hands. Do this ten times, then repeat the strokes on the other side.

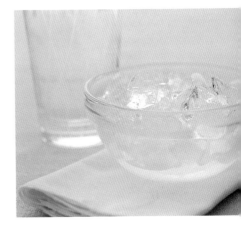

Keep the Water Coming
Always drink plenty of water after receiving a cross-fiber massage to flush away any newly released toxins. And if an area of your body is very sore, ice it for seven to ten minutes before and after the massage.

laughter therapy

Whether it's a chuckle, a guffaw, or a fit of the giggles, laughter does more than just make you feel good: It boosts your immunity and makes your heart stronger.

Why Can't You Tickle Yourself?
Go ahead, try. Even if you tickle yourself in the exact same spot and in the exact same way that makes you hysterical when someone else does it to you, you won't produce even a tiny giggle, much less a guffaw. Researchers speculate that while the information sent to your central nervous system should be identical, the crucial elements of tension and surprise are missing.

"The earth laughs in flowers," poet and philosopher Ralph Waldo Emerson wrote more than a century ago, and, indeed, laughter is a beautiful thing. It brings a twinkle to your eye and a flush to your cheek, and the sound of it makes people all around start to smile. It's also good for your health: When you laugh, the level of stress hormones in your body goes down and you produce more of the cells and proteins that attack viruses, tumors, and harmful bacteria. Laughter also enhances the flow and oxygenation of blood, which is invigorating and aids healing. It's even a form of exercise, providing a workout for muscles in your face, chest, back, and abdomen.

If you're having trouble seeing the lighter side of life, there are humor programs offered worldwide—at hospitals, schools, corporations, and senior centers. You can, in fact, find laughter clubs that specialize in stimulating the sillies in groups of people. That approach might sound forced, but workshop leaders swear that sometimes people just need a little guidance to get the giggles going—and once the merriment starts, greater health and deeper friendships are sure to follow.

THE ANATOMY OF LAUGHTER

Neurobiologists have found that all laughter consists of clipped, vowel-like sounds (such as ha-ha) repeated every 210 milliseconds. Laughter causes more than a dozen facial muscles to contract, including the one that's primarily responsible for lifting your upper lip. Your epiglottis (thin cartilage that protects the space between the vocal cords) partly closes up your larynx (the upper entrance to the windpipe), making you gasp for air. When you're *really* tickled, your tear ducts react, producing streams of joyful tears.

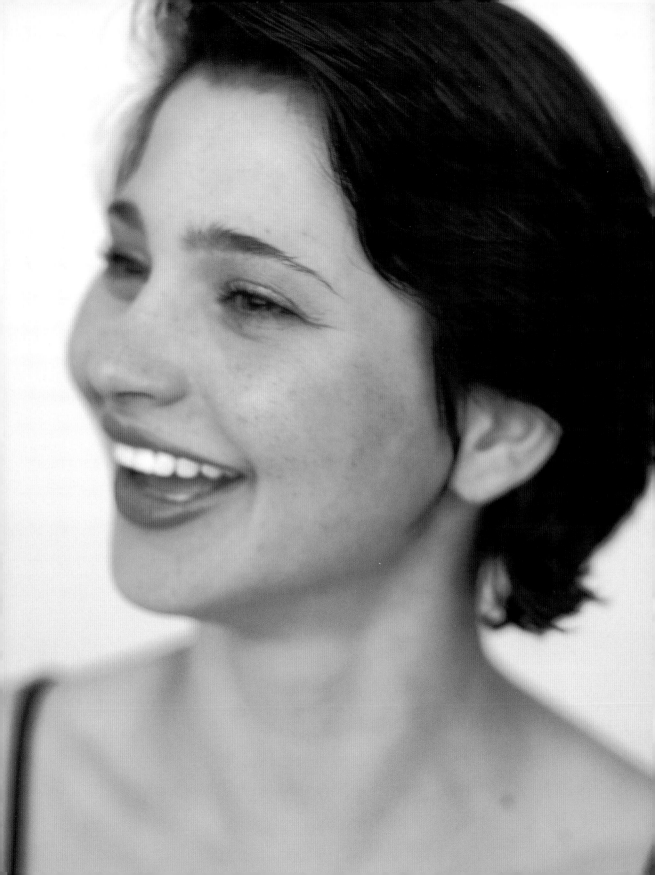

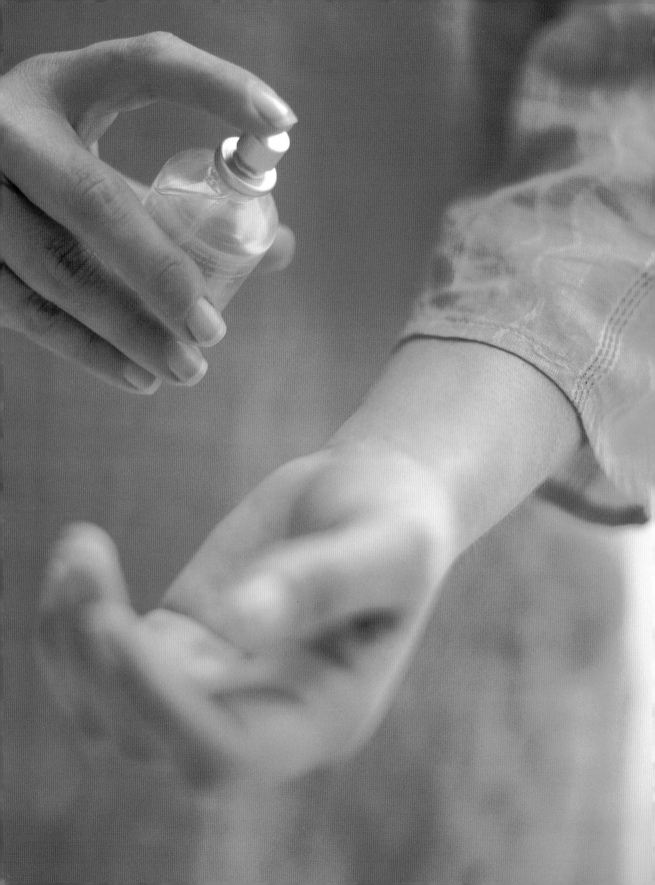

signature scents

No need to try on every cologne, hoping to find one that suits you. A new crop of mix-and-match fragrances makes it easy to create your own unique blend.

When you're on a quest to find that perfect new perfume or cologne, spraying on dozens of testers at the store can result in olfactory overload and a cacophony of clashing scents. The scents can seem too sweetly floral, too spicy, too woodsy, or just plain too-too. But now, recognizing the highly individualistic nature of our sense of smell, several manufacturers are offering lines of colognes that are meant to be blended or layered, allowing each customer to create her own signature scent—one that can be easily altered to suit her mood, the time of day, or even the occasion.

Some of the blendables are simple, single-note fragrances, while others are more complex fragrances with a blend of top, middle, and base notes. In the lingo of perfumers, the top note is your first impression, the middle note appears after a perfume has had a chance to dry and different essences have expanded, and the base note is the scent that will linger long into the day. Make sure that you find all the notes in your personal blend harmonious.

To find the perfect scent for you, mix various combinations of fragrances on a sheet of paper, rather than directly on your wrist. (You can discard the paper if you don't like the results—an option that's easier than repeatedly washing your arm.) When you think you've devised a pleasing blend, then it's time to try it out on your skin. This is a crucial step: The fragrance will change as it reacts to the levels of acidity and oiliness of your skin—that's why the same perfume can smell different on other people. To apply, spray on a light mist of one scent. Then layer on one or more other scents until you've re-created the blend that smelled good to you on paper. To be sure that you've hit upon a winning combination, leave the fragrance on for a while and notice how it smells as time passes.

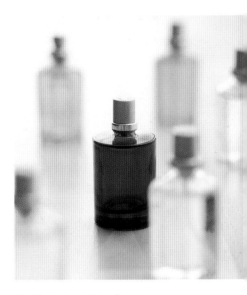

The Myth about Pulse Points
Pay no heed to the advice about dabbing fragrance on pulse points; research has shown that this has a negligible effect on its dispersion. French fashion diva Coco Chanel offered much wiser counsel: She simply suggested that women put perfume wherever they want to be kissed.

glossary

acupressure A healing massage technique that uses thumb or fingertip pressure to stimulate acupuncture points.

acupuncture A 6,000-year-old Chinese healing tradition that involves placing needles into the skin at specific points to balance the flow of *chi* and treat illnesses.

antioxidant A molecule that suppresses various effects of oxidation and in particular free radicals, especially the short-lived, highly reactive oxygen types.

aromatherapy The skilled use of essential oils to promote physical, emotional, and spiritual wellbeing. The essential oils may be heated, dropped into baths, or applied (in a diluted form) to the skin.

aromatic oil See essential oil.

asana The Sanskrit term for a yoga pose. *Asanas* are designed to improve physical, spiritual, and emotional health.

astringent See toner.

Ayurveda The traditional medicine of India. This holistic health-care system teaches that each person has a core of peace and perfection—a natural state of wellbeing and happiness. Ayurvedic practices help people return to this natural state by balancing their life energies and helping them achieve harmony with the environment.

Bikram yoga A modern form of yoga that consists of 26 poses practiced in hot rooms to promote detoxification.

bromelain An enzyme that aids digestion. It's found in foods such as pineapple.

calorie A unit of measurement used in some countries to describe how much energy a food item has. Multiply calories by 4.186 for the equivalent in kilojoules.

carbohydrates Carbohydrates are essentially sugar and starch; when used as energy, they become fuel for our muscles and brain. They can be found in foods such as bread, grains, potatoes, apples, oranges, and candy.

carpal tunnel syndrome A condition in which the nerve in the wrist becomes compressed (often by repetitive motion) and causes weakness and pain.

carrier oil An inert oil (usually vegetable or mineral) used to hold or dilute more potent substances such as essential oils. A carrier oil is generally used to reduce the concentration of a substance, making it safe for use on the skin.

cellulite Subcutaneous fat with a pitted appearance, much like an orange peel.

chakra Translated as "wheel" in Sanskrit, a *chakra* is a point through which energy enters and leaves the body. Eastern traditions believe that the body has seven chakras, each associated with certain mental or emotional characteristics.

chi In Chinese medicine, *chi* is the vital life energy that flows through the body (and the universe). Chinese healers believe that blockages or deficiencies of chi are the root cause of disease.

cholesterol A waxy fat that comes both from the liver and from foods we eat, especially meat and dairy products. Nutritionists divide cholesterol into two groups: HDL cholesterol, which is considered "good," and LDL cholesterol, which is considered "bad," or unhealthful.

citronella oil An essential oil that is known for its bug-repelling properties.

collagen The main protein in connective tissue. Collagen lends skin its strength. The degradation of collagen is a cause of the formation of wrinkles.

comedogenic Describes a substance that can cause or worsen pimples, blackheads, and whiteheads (to identify products intended to discourage these types of skin problems, look for the term *non-comedogenic* on product labels).

conditioner A substance designed to restore the healthy look of hair, which may have been damaged by excessive heat, chemical processes, or rough handling.

dietary fiber The bulky part of food (generally plants) that cannot be broken down by enzymes in the digestive system. Fiber helps move food through the intestines faster, and its consumption has been linked to decreased rates of cancer.

diffuser A device that distributes (often via heat) the aroma from an essential oil.

diuretic Any substance that increases the amount of urine the body produces.

elastin A protein that makes skin elastic.

ellagic acid A phytochemical with strong antioxidant and antibacterial properties. It's found in foods such as strawberries.

endocrine system The system of glands that produce various chemical secretions (hormones) that circulate, via the blood, throughout the body.

essential oil An oil that gives plants their characteristic odor. These oils are used for aromatherapy, as well as in perfumery.

exfoliant A grainy scrub agent designed to help clear skin of its residual dead cells.

exfoliate To scrub off dead skin cells.

fats Organic compounds that make up the most concentrated source of energy in food. *Total fat* measures all types of fat in a food. *Saturated fat* measures only the amount of a specific type of fat, which is the biggest dietary source of high LDL levels (or "bad" cholesterol).

free radicals Unstable molecules that have been linked to the degeneration of human biological functions. Free radicals are thought to contribute to disorders such as heart disease and cancer.

glutes The nickname for the *glutei maximi*, the muscles in the buttocks.

hamstrings The long muscles that run along the back of the thighs.

hatha yoga A form of yoga that combines postures and breathing exercises to balance the body's energies. The word *hatha* comes from the Sanskrit words *ha* (sun) and *tha* (moon); the goal of the practice is to unite and balance solar (energizing) and lunar (relaxing) energies.

heart chakra The "energy center" in the heart; this chakra is associated with love and generosity (see chakra).

heliotrope A plant with fragrant flowers ranging in color from violet to white.

kilojoule A unit of measurement used internationally to describe how much energy a food item has. Divide kilojoules by 4.186 for the equivalent in calories.

kosher salt A refined yet coarse-grained salt that contains no additives (it's called kosher because it is used to make meat kosher by drawing out the blood).

labyrinth A network of passages or paths, all leading to one central spot.

lactic acid A by-product of a process that delivers energy to muscles when they demand more oxygen than the blood can deliver. Lactic acid can cause a burning sensation during vigorous exercise.

loofah A rough sponge that is made from the dried pod of a gourd and is a good tool to use for exfoliating skin.

lymphatic system A network of spaces between body tissues and organs through which lymph (a pale fluid that has white blood cells in it) circulates.

melanin A naturally occurring dark pigment that is found in the skin or hair. When we're exposed to sunlight, our skin darkens because the skin produces more melanin.

meridian In Chinese medicine, a channel or path in the body through which energy (or *chi*) travels. Acupuncture points are located along the meridians; stimulating those points helps balance the flow of chi along that meridian.

metabolic waste The normal waste products that the body makes in the course of its day-to-day functioning.

moisturizer A substance or product that reduces moisture loss from the skin.

nadis Sometimes translated as "conduits," "nerves," or "vessels," Ayurvedic nadis—like Chinese meridians—are the channels through which life energy flows.

neroli oil Produced from the white blossoms of the bitter or Seville orange tree, neroli oil (also called orange blossom oil) exudes an aroma that aromatherapists

say can help calm emotions, as well as help promote restful sleep.

neurotransmitter A substance that transmits impulses between nerve cells.

orrisroot Derived from the roots of iris plants, it is used as a fixative (or fragrance preservative) in perfumes and elsewhere.

osteoporosis A syndrome in which the bones become less dense, more brittle, and prone to breakage.

phenols A category of phytochemicals, including the compounds that make berries blue and eggplants violet. Phenols are potent antioxidants with anticlotting and anti-inflammatory properties.

phytochemicals Plant chemicals. Some phytochemicals have been reported to fight or protect against many diseases, ward off cell damage, stimulate the immune system, and aid the body's detoxification mechanisms.

Pilates A system of exercises developed by the German dancer and boxer Joseph Pilates in the 1920s. Pilates exercises strengthen and elongate muscles, thus improving posture and flexibility.

polyphenols A type of phenols found in substances such as wine, coffee, and tea. Polyphenols are potent antioxidants.

pores The openings to the sweat gland tubes on the surface of the skin. Sweat glands secrete perspiration and help regulate body temperature.

prana The Sanskrit word for life force.

pranayama Yogic breathing exercises designed to increase *prana*, or life force.

proteins Complex organic compounds made up of amino acids that supply the body with energy and enable functions such as building tissue. Food sources that are high in protein include meat, dairy products, grains, and legumes.

pumice stone A very light and porous volcanic rock that can be used to scrub off rough skin, especially on the feet.

quads (quadriceps) The muscles that run along the front of the thighs.

reflexology A type of massage that involves applying pressure to specific points on the hands and feet based on the belief that this pressure can benefit other body parts.

repetitive-stress injury An injury to cartilage, tendons, ligaments, nerves, or muscles that results from doing the same physical motion repeatedly.

Sanskrit An ancient language in India that is used in academia and religion—much like Latin is used in Western countries.

scrub A product designed to exfoliate dead skin cells that contains small granules.

self-tanning lotion A product containing dihydroxyacetone (DHA) that reacts with amino acids in the uppermost skin layers to trigger melanin-producing cells and make the skin look tanned.

Spleen 16 An acupressure point, at the base of the rib cage directly below each nipple, used to relieve indigestion, nausea, and abdominal cramps, and to balance the appetite and gastrointestinal system.

T-zone The forehead, nose, and chin on the human face, which tend to be oilier than other areas of the face.

tai chi An ancient Chinese fighting and healing tradition that consists of slow, graceful movements designed to balance and strengthen the body's *chi*, or energy.

terpenes A category of phytochemicals found in foods ranging from spinach to soy. Terpenes are powerful antioxidants.

thymus gland A ductless gland in the throat area that aids the immune system.

toner Also called astringent or freshener. A facial cleansing product that removes residual traces of make-up, oil, and other impurities. Toner has a refreshing and cooling action on the skin. It also can temporarily make pores look smaller.

yoga An ancient Indian system that combines *asanas* (poses) with *pranayama* (breathing) and meditation. The goal of yoga is to enhance physical, emotional, and spiritual health.

yogi One who practices yoga.

index

acknowledgments

We wish to thank the following people for their generous assistance in producing this book: Additional photography by Sheri Giblin, pages 41, 45, 63, 109, 126, 128, 141, 175, 187, 234–35, 250, 261, and 310; Quentin Bacon, pages 171 and 216; Maren Caruso, pages 265 and 291; Beatriz da Costa, page 49; Rhonda J. Kist, page 12; David Loftus, pages 170, 267, and 289; Valerie Martin, page 148; William Meppem, pages 74, 99, 214, 247, and 298; Minh & Wass, pages 23 (top right) and 70; Amy Neunsinger, page 238; and Caroline Schiff, page 313. Joanna Brown, The Body Shop's global product manager for accessories, who was tremendously helpful; Jennie Laar, The Body Shop's global product manager for gifts; Claudia Hackett, The Body Shop's copy approval manager, who made many valuable contributions; Susie Flook, The Body Shop's group general counsel; photography assistants Keith Hutter and Brandon McGanty; Blue Sky Rental Studios; stylist Karen Young; Robin Terra, Terra Studios, for assistance with preliminary design concepts; Jackie Mancuso and Efrat Rafaeli for design assistance; Marc Ericksen for illustrations; Kathy Schermerhorn for color management; Laura Schlieske for tai chi consultations; Kristine Ravn for assistance with international relations; Emily Jahn for all of her support; Maria Behan for creative writing; Julianne Balmain for marketing copy; Sunah Cherwin and Gail Nelson-Bonebrake for proofreading; models Aubri Balk, Scott Blossom, Bree Blumstein, Rebecca Chang, Sarah Coleman, Helen Demuth, Jennifer "Lexi" Durst, Chandra Easton, Timothy Floreen, Michelle Gagnon, Nicole Ganas, Neha Gheewala, Elena Grassel, Rebecca Handler, Kristie Dahlia Home, Brandon McGanty, Alisha Meek, Lulu Monti, Ryan Mortensen, Athena Pappas, Mia Parler, Carmen Peirano, Justine Roddick, Maiya Roddick-Fuller, Monica Roseberry, Kristin Rostek, Rachel Ruperto, Laura Schlieske, Ramona Schwarz, Angella Sprauve, Randy Stanley, Heather Tomilin, Lea Watkins, Cynthia R. Wren, Crystal Wright, Liz Yee, Alicia Dunams Youngson, and Lake Ziwa-Rodriguez.

⬭ **THE BODY SHOP**

Save **20%**
on any Aromatherapy
body-care purchase
with this coupon

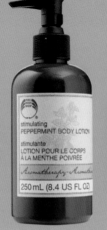

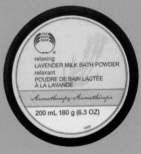

Wash on a new mood with Aromatherapy
body wash, body salt scrub, body lotion,
and massage oil. Available in Stimulating
Peppermint, Relaxing Lavender, Sensual
Ylang Ylang, and Energizing Bergamot.